Dedicated to Hope

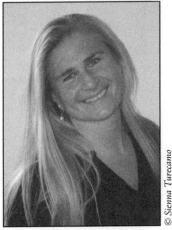

© Sienna Turecamo

About the Author

Nathalie W. Herrman (Virginia) is a personal trainer, motivational speaker, massage therapist, and Reiki master. She graduated magna cum laude from Boston University and has spent her life accumulating experience in the pursuit of optimal health and wellness in herself and others. Visit her online at www.nathaliewherrman.com.

THE ART OF GOOD HABITS

Health, Love, Presence & Prosperity

NATHALIE W. HERRMAN

Llewellyn Publications
Woodbury, Minnesota

FIRST EDITION
First Printing, 2015

Book design: Bob Gaul
Cover art: iStockphoto.com/4658396/©emrah_oztas
iStockphoto.com/13205999/©samxmeg
iStockphoto.com/19353220/©pepifoto
iStockphoto.com/3543943/©pappamaart
iStockphoto.com/8370796/©Dole08
iStockphoto.om/323006/©sx70
Part Page art: iStockphoto.om/323006/©sx70
Cover design: Ellen Lawson
Editing: Ed Day

Llewellyn Publications is a registered trademark of Llewellyn Worldwide Ltd.

Library of Congress Cataloging-in-Publication Data
Herrman, Nathalie W.
  The art of good habits: health, love, presence & prosperity/Nathalie W. Herrman.—First
Edition.   pages cm
  ISBN 978-0-7387-4600-5
1. Well-being. I. Title.
  BD431.H4519 2015
  650.1—dc23
                        2015029970

Llewellyn Publications, a Division of Llewellyn Worldwide Ltd.
2143 Wooddale Drive
Woodbury, MN 55125-2989
www.llewellyn.com
Printed in the United States of America

Acknowledgments

"Silent Gratitude isn't much use to anyone."
—G. B. Stern

I would like to thank Angela Wix for being my guiding light on this project. I couldn't have done it without her vision and unending support. And everyone at Llewellyn for their willingness to bring *The Art of Good Habits* to life. And my husband, Gruff, for his steady love, his ready availability to discuss all kinds of ideas and philosophical musings that were sparked by my writing, and his Herculean trust in the work. This has been an enlightening and invaluable process for me, and I am deeply grateful and forever changed by the fascinating experience of authoring this book.

Disclaimer

This book is not intended to provide medical advice or to take the place of medical advice and treatment from your personal physician. Readers are advised to consult their doctors or other qualified health-care professionals regarding the treatment of their medical problems. Neither the publisher nor the author take any responsibility for any possible consequences from any treatment, action, or application to any person reading or following the information in this book.

Contents

Introduction   1

PART ONE: HEALTH   9

....

**Chapter One: Honesty, Awareness,
Attitude, and Food   13**

Keeping an Open Mind   19

How We Feel about Ourselves and the Way We Eat   23

What We Know: The Practical Facts   31

More Practicality: Fats, Carbs, and Sugar   34

Understanding Hunger and the
Importance of Accountability   38

Believing We're Worth It   45

**Chapter Two: Turning Honesty
into Health as a Habit 49**

Planning Carefully 54

Being Prepared at Home 59

Eating Mindfully 62

The Voice that Tells Us When 66

To Weigh or Not To Weigh 69

Movement as a Spiritual Practice 71

The Basics of Exercise 74

Body Love 80

The Importance of Sleep 85

Review and Daily Action Plan 85

PART TWO: LOVE 87

....

**Chapter Three: Authenticity,
Willingness, and Compassion 91**

In the Beginning 98

Expectations Versus Reality 101

Potential and Discernment 105

Compassion and Appreciation 108

Authenticity 110

Identifying Blocks 113

The Drawbridge of Love 114

Accepting Ourselves as We Are 116

Chapter Four: Turning Willingness into Love as a Habit 121

Taking Responsibility 123

Forgiveness 124

Intimate Relationships 129

Simple but Not Easy: The Importance of Boundaries 134

Review and Daily Action Plan 139

PART THREE: PRESENCE 141

Chapter Five: Awareness and the Purpose of Time 145

How Attitude Affects Our Experience 152

Time as a Gift 155

Why We're Not Present 157

Pleasure in the Mix 161

What Blocks Us? 162

Regarding Habitual Lateness 166

Time as It Is 168

Chapter Six: Turning Awareness into Presence as a Habit 173

Preparation and Organization 174

Aligning with Our Natural Rhythms 177

Making Adjustments and Eliminating the Unnecessary 181

The Choice Is Ours   190

Aging Gracefully   192

Review and Daily Action Plan   195

PART FOUR: PROSPERITY   197

Chapter Seven: Fear, Appreciation, and the Abundance Mindset   201

Appreciation   207

Measuring Values and the Principle of Abundance   211

Beyond the Material   213

The Big Picture   214

Discipline and Commitment   219

Chapter Eight: Turning Appreciation Into Prosperity as a Habit   223

The Benefits of Generosity   231

Gratitude   236

Gratitude in Action   241

Review and Daily Action Plan   244

Conclusion   247

Exercise List

Part One: Health 9

Honesty Exercise: Self-Discovery   16

Awareness Exercise: Learning to Tune In   21

Honesty Exercise: Where to Begin   28

Honesty Exercise: What We Are
Actually Eating, and Why?   42

Willingness Exercise: Affirmations
to Create Momentum   46

Awareness Exercise: Eating Mindfully Meditation   64

Awareness Exercise: Learning to
Listen to the Voice Within   68

Willingness Exercise: Movement   76

Appreciation Exercise: Your Body, Your Friend   82

Part Two: Love   87

Honesty Exercise: Where You
Stand with Relationships   92

Awareness Exercise: Expectations
and What You Believe   104

Willingness Exercise: Embracing
Your Authentic Self   111

Awareness Exercise: Opening to Love   115

Appreciation Exercise: Compassion for Others   118

Willingness Exercise: Visualization
for Becoming Courageous   122

Willingness Exercise: Catching Yourself   127

Willingness Exercise: Daily
Practice for Growing Love   132

Appreciation Exercise: Visualization
for Healthy Boundaries   137

Part Three: Presence   141

Honesty Exercise: How Do You Spend Your Time?   149

Awareness Exercise: Doing and Being Meditation   154

Awareness Exercise: Discovering What Matters   159

Willingness Exercise: Letting Go of Blocks   164

Willingness Exercise: Committing to Change   169

Willingness Exercise: Technology Detox   176

Appreciation Exercise: Daily Practice
for Observing Rhythms   179

Awareness Exercise: Daily Checklist
for Establishing Boundaries   185

Appreciation Exercise: Self-Evolution Visualization   194

Part Four: Prosperity   197

Honesty Exercise: What Are You Afraid Of?   203

Appreciation Exercise: Less Is More Visualization   208

Appreciation Exercise: Understanding Values   212

Honesty Exercise: Creating a Mission Statement   217

Willingness Exercise: Committing to Abundance   221

Awareness and Willingness Exercise:
Identifying and Eliminating Physical Clutter   225

Awareness Exercise: Generosity Checklist   234

Appreciation Exercise: Daily Gratitude List   239

Appreciation Exercise: Caring for Our Lives   243

Introduction

"Let perseverance be your engine and hope your fuel."
—H. Jackson Brown, Jr.

I have come to believe, and believe powerfully, that when we are willing to take responsibility for changing ourselves, we become unlimited in potential. We have the ability to improve by gradual degrees in any direction we choose for as long as we live. And everything that happens can be something to grow us and evolve us and raise us to the next level of understanding and contentment and the next.

The trouble with not accepting responsibility for ourselves is that we feel helpless, and that makes us grabby and greedy. It empowers the "more" mentality. We don't realize our ability to be patient and trusting, so we push to the front and demand our share first, or demand more than our share. And the people we meet on this path are doing the same thing. We are all pushing and grabbing and trying to get there first, wherever "there" might be.

When we act this way, we have no faith in time, no faith in there being enough, and no faith in *our* being enough. We are empty and crazy with lust. Our wants are urgent, and we don't care who we hurt in order to satisfy them. But by maintaining this mindset, we entirely miss the point, and our dissatisfaction becomes a vicious cycle. We grab for as much as we can get, and in so doing, we show no love and compassion for others. And maybe we spend money that we don't have to try to change our internal feelings of isolation, or maybe we overeat, or maybe we bounce from one empty intimate relationship to another. All this because we refuse to own the divine spark within us and the power of our own light. As a result, our problems are largely the product of our not believing in our own wholeness and lacking faith in our ability to step up and take responsibility for the condition of our lives.

We are famously good at the blame game. We blame our parents, our upbringing, our jobs, and our bosses. We blame our financial condition. We blame our ex-husbands, ex-wives, current husbands, and current wives. We blame our third-grade teacher and our old friend. We blame our digestion, the traffic, the weather—anything will do as long as it takes the responsibility off of us. We point the finger and create imaginary distance. These are the things responsible for our dissatisfaction. If only they were different, we would be happy. Our unhappiness is their fault. Or is it?

Perhaps not. Perhaps, our unhappiness exists primarily inside of us—in our perspective, our attitude, and our system of beliefs. And if that's the case, that's good news, because these are things we have the power to change! This is the thinking behind this book. My hope is to empower you as the reader to claim your happiness by changing what's not working in your life. It can be done by making adjustments in your habits and your point of view.

I have learned this from my own experience. As a young adult, I struggled with addictive and compulsive behaviors. I was "grabby" to the extreme. I turned to anything and everything to make me happy; sometimes I would get a burst of temporary euphoria, but nothing that I landed upon ever kept me happy. I was in a cycle of constantly seeking, and I was empty on the inside.

Eventually, I reached an emotional and physical bottom. My craving and grasping led me to bankruptcy on every level, and my life was out of control. I came to a point where I had to get honest and become willing to make changes, or self-destruct by default. I had a choice: a defining moment. I could step out of denial and take ownership of my mess and begin to climb out of the mire, or I could continue to spiral downward. With courage and guidance, I chose to get honest. And that has changed everything.

But honesty is uncomfortable. I had to look at my darkness. I had to look at my dysfunction, and dis-ease, and the layer upon layer of my self-limiting beliefs. It was the most difficult thing I have ever had to do because my ego could no longer protect me.

I was completely undraped. No pretense was left and no pretense was possible. I was raw and vulnerable and willing to change. And in this tender state, I was unexpectedly set free from all falsehood. I was as I was: imperfect, but not alone. I came to understand that others who had gone before me and were a bit farther down the path could help me find my way. And just as others were there to guide me, I hope that this book may serve as a guide to you.

I believe that the process of self-discovery is the most important work that we have in this lifetime. Embarking on this journey can be unsettling and is no easy task, but I also believe that in the end, what we discover will not be some dark and scary apparition, but a being of pure light and pure love. That's who we are. And yet, our fear of the unknown keeps us trapped behind a veil of our own making. We are shielded from our glory. We let our misperceptions, our coping mechanisms, and our unhealthy habits define us.

This book is for those who have the courage to look behind the veil, explore the depths of their own being, and live their best life—not some compromised, settled-for existence, but a shining and glorious vibrant life! This does not come without effort. It requires a mindset that believes in what's possible, a willingness to be honest, and the courage to change. Enlightened living requires persistence, diligence, and self-reflection. If you want to be free from what limits you, I encourage you to make the decision now to do whatever it takes.

I have been a personal trainer and massage therapist for fifteen years, and I have worked with all kinds of people with all kinds of attitudes. I have worked with their bodies, their diets, and their challenges in life. I have both witnessed and experienced self-defeat, pride, false humility, and fear in every form. And equally so, I have witnessed and experienced absolute authenticity, courage, and the power of love. I have been privy to incredible change and growth in some of my clients, and stagnation and a kind of flatline maintenance of the status quo in others. The difference is in people's attitudes, their beliefs, and their willingness to take action. This book and this journey are not for the skeptical and the cynical; they are for those who aren't afraid to do the work that it takes to evolve.

The Art of Good Habits is built on the pillars of four spiritual principles: honesty, willingness, awareness, and appreciation. And while each of these has applications across the board in regard to our well-being, one more than the other is associated with each main topic. Developing good habits in relation to our health is primarily linked to our ability to be honest, our experience of love has to do with our level of willingness, our experience of presence is affiliated with awareness, and prosperity comes from appreciation.

The order of the main topics follows the same direction of each chapter and of the book's larger purpose, making a kind of progression within a progression like a stack of Russian nesting dolls. To change habits, there is an evolutionary pathway that starts with honesty, moves through willingness and awareness, and ends in appreciation. You will notice that each exercise is connected to one of these principles and that the first one in each section is honesty, and the last one is appreciation. My thesis throughout is that by using these principles in the manner suggested, you can come to enjoy a sense of empowerment and control over challenging issues in your life.

Consequently, if you fully make this book your own, participate in the exercises, and actively involve yourself in the process of reading, considering, and self-reflecting, you will benefit the most. *The Art of Good Habits* is not designed as entertainment, although it may be entertaining. It is designed for guidance, a kind of road map to wellness and life satisfaction. But looking at a map is not the same thing as using one. Even a GPS system doesn't do much good if we hear what's being said but don't follow the cue.

I encourage you to read with a pen in your hand. Underline, take notes, scribble in the columns, and do the exercises! Or, if you prefer, do all of that electronically, but involve yourself beyond the act of simply reading the words. The point is to find a way to integrate the suggested concepts into your actual life circumstances so that you can reap the benefits. This book has a purpose, and the purpose is for you as the reader to feel better than you ever thought possible. It's simple, but not easy, to raise your awareness, overcome your limiting beliefs, and embrace the wealth that you carry within.

Ours is a vital role—the most vital role—in the level of happiness that we experience. It requires a particular attitude, and does not come from having the perfect body, the ideal lover, or a winning lottery ticket. Being happy or unhappy doesn't depend on how effectively we race against time, or how much we accomplish. It is the result of having respect for what matters and demonstrating that effectively in our behavior and in our approach to life.

This is the beginning of a journey through health, love, presence, and prosperity. It involves the application of skill and creative imagination, the merging of the practical with the divine, and the reconciling of spiritual principles with concrete action steps. This is *The Art of Good Habits*. I invite you to turn the page, and open your mind.

PART ONE

·····················

HEALTH

"Behold yourself."
—Deepak Chopra

This section of the book, "Health," is divided into two chapters. The first chapter, "Honesty, Awareness, Attitude, and Food," establishes a kind of playing field, or setting. Through discussion and suggested exercises, we bring awareness to where we are in our lives in relation to our health. We look around, and get honest. We consider how we got to the place we currently find ourselves and determine if we're happy being there or if we want something better—if, in fact, we believe that we deserve something better. We get quiet and focus within. We consider what our goals are going forward and in what direction we might want to move.

In chapter two, "Turning Honesty into Health as a Habit," we get moving, literally. We take steps to change the way we experience our body, our health, and our well-being. We create new patterns of behavior to improve the quality of our daily experience and consider the role that exercise plays in our lives. We find the spiritual basis for maintaining an open mind, for physical movement, for eating with care, and for a good night's sleep. We begin with health because it is the most obvious place where our habits show up, and by making appropriate changes in this regard, we see immediate positive results.

CHAPTER ONE

· · · · · · · · · · · · · · · · · · · ·

Honesty, Awareness, Attitude, and Food

"A light supper, a good night's sleep, and a fine
morning have often made a hero of the same man,
who, by indigestion, a restless night, and a rainy
morning, would have proved a coward."
—Chesterfield

Health is a vast topic about which volumes could be, and have,
been written. I am not a doctor and am not qualified to write
prescriptions. I am, however, qualified to share my perspective
and my experience. Having worked in the health and fitness in-
dustry for more than fifteen years and taken my own journey on
the healing path, my perspective has its application, particularly
as it relates to the specific focus of this book.

There is much about our health that we have very little control over: our genetic makeup, susceptibility and sensitivity to allergies, chemical imbalance, athleticism and coordination, and a whole host of additional factors and disorders of a physical nature. But we do have the ability to control some elements of our health—our attitude and the way we eat being primary among them—and these will be the focus of this chapter.

Generally speaking, many of us tend to take an all-or-nothing approach to self-improvement. We get "on track" for a while, and then somehow, without even understanding why it happens, we become completely derailed. We are upbeat and positive, willing and eager; we make good food choices, and then, with a kind of righteous indignation, we say forget it, and overindulge our food and our moods to the extreme. But flip-flopping back and forth like this is not conducive to feeling good. What feels good, over time, is a steady and sustainable balance.

But balance is less obvious than it seems. It is not a perfect stance where all is equal. It requires constant adjustments and continuous focus. Think of a man on a tightrope. He is never still. Even when he is not moving forward, he is shifting his arms and bending his knees and making small changes in his position at all times in order to stay upright and stay centered and stay "in balance." I know this from my work at the gym as well. Increasing our ability to balance requires that we risk a little discomfort by making ourselves temporarily unstable. We feel shaky and unsure. We wobble back and forth as we try to stand on a round and squishy surface or on one foot or whatever the exercise might be. And we want to get back on solid ground.

The only way to improve our balance is to allow for this unsteadiness. We practice in short spurts. We wobble for ten seconds the first day, and twenty the next. We learn to become slightly more comfortable with the instability and the constant positional adjustment that is required. We slowly build new stabilizing muscles. And before long, we are able to stand comfortably for a long period of time on the unsteady surface and perform all manner of movement. And then we up the ante. We increase the challenge to the next level and the next, and our balance gets better every time. That's the way it works at the gym, and that's the way it works in life.

We won't make any effort to improve our balance, however, if we have no knowledge that it needs improving in the first place, so self-honesty comes first. We have to admit that we have imbalances and dissatisfaction in life before we can start the work of making things better for ourselves. But self-honesty, like balance, is a bit tricky. Our thinking is cluttered with projection, nostalgia, and complaining, so that's what we hear, and that's what guides us. But if we can learn to disseminate the wheat from the chaff, so to speak, and the clutter from the facts, then everything becomes simpler, and we know exactly what we're dealing with and exactly where to begin.

Honesty Exercise: Self-Discovery

This exercise will guide you to personal truth through a process of reduction and simplification. You will begin with a mass of thought; consider it, and pare it down until you arrive at essential self-honesty. You will need a pen or a pencil, a journal of some kind (that you may continue to use throughout the book), and a few minutes of quiet, uninterrupted time. If you prefer to do your journaling online, you can use your computer or iPad. The use of the term "journal" going forth will refer to whatever method you choose. The exercise requires that you write three statements:

+ The first can be multiple sentences and have some detail about what you tell yourself in relation to the challenges you face regarding one particular aspect of your diet or your attitude toward life.

+ The second is restating the same thing in a simpler way—two sentences max.

+ And the third is restating it again in the simplest way possible—one short sentence—minus all projection and excuses and complaining and fluff.

EXAMPLE #1

+ I don't have time to eat well. I'm not a morning person, so I can't be bothered with breakfast. I grab something quick on the way to work—a coffee and Danish maybe, or a protein bar. And I hardly ever have time for lunch, so I usually skip it, and just snack on whatever's in the break-room. And after work I usually get takeout because it's easy and I'm tired. And then I munch on whatever I can find at night while I'm watching TV.

- I eat for convenience. I grab breakfast on the run, skip lunch, and eat whatever for dinner. I eat mindlessly, like I don't really care. But I do care...

- *I don't eat well.*

Once we have our statement reduced to this simple form, we have something we can work with. This is self-honesty! This is where we can begin!

EXAMPLE #2

- I have tried lots of diets, but none of them have worked for me. One time I lost fifteen pounds, but I gained it back. I really don't understand why I struggle with my weight the way I do because I usually pay attention to what I eat. I think my diet is pretty healthy. The fact that I'm as heavy as I am frustrates me. It doesn't seem fair.

- I feel like I eat well, but I'm still struggling with my weight.

- *I am struggling with my weight.*

Ah, so simple. We can work with this. This is what we're after. This is self-honesty.

Example #3

+ I am mostly healthy, but I am afraid of getting sick or getting injured. I worry a lot about my joints and my back, and I'm always trying to be careful with them. And what if I get cancer or something like that? I worry about that. And I worry about the health of my family as well. I am stressed out a lot and I don't sleep well and I drink more than I should and I'm a little overweight.

+ I am afraid of getting sick or someone I love getting sick. And I worry a lot, too, which causes me stress.

+ *I worry a lot.*

Again! This is a workable place to start. We can deal with this as a simple statement of fact.

The point here is that reducing our voluminous thoughts down to their essential truths helps us to know what we're really dealing with, and then things become more manageable. Now, take a few minutes to write down your own three statements. Don't overthink it.

1. In your journal, write a few sentences about the way you feel challenged in regard to food, or the way you feel frustrated with life in general.

2. Now, rewrite what you have written above, but simplify it some. Eliminate anything that seems non-essential (refer to the examples above if you're not sure how to do this).

3. One more time, rewrite what you have written above. But this time, reduce it to its absolute simplest form (refer to the examples above for guidance). This statement that you have written represents a "truth" in your life.

What we learn from this exercise is something about the nature of self-honesty and the nature of self-deception as well. It's easy and natural to fog ourselves in with convoluted thinking. More often than not, this thinking is riddled with fear about the future—all the things that could go wrong and all the reasons that something won't work out for us. And that's what we come to believe about the way things are. But once we clearly understand what's actually at play—that kernel of truth is in the mass of our thinking—we realize that we have the power to change our thinking, change our behavior, and consequently experience the results of better choices in our lives.

Keeping an Open Mind

Our mental outlook plays no small role in the state of our health. It contributes greatly to our sense of well-being, or lack thereof. We are all familiar with concepts of optimism and negativity, and perhaps we identify ourselves with one camp more than the other.

But I would argue that they both have their limitations—they are both "skewed" in one direction or the other—tilted east and west.

The healthiest mental approach to life may well be found in neutrality, which allows for the appreciation of things "as they are," unaffected by our wanting them or expecting them to be good or bad. We readily become psychologically fixed on projections of the future in a kind of advanced certainty. We expect things to be either positive or disastrous, and we worry about and prepare for situations that never actually come to pass. We spend endless hours thinking and thinking and thinking. Our thoughts spiral and flip.

We wake up and our minds go straight to work, solving the potential problems of the day, wondering and worrying about the people we may encounter, the things we have to do, and all that could go wrong, or right. We fret and scheme and ponder and figure. We calculate and delegate. We create mock conversations and arguments and have speeches prepared in advance should we need them for any reason. And all the while, life is happening, and we are missing it, lost in our heads.

Learning the nature of our minds is important spiritual work. It is spiritual as well as mental; it consists of both thinking and letting go of thinking. Our minds will control us, and not necessarily in a beneficial way, unless we learn to control them. And we learn to control our minds through the practice of self-honesty as demonstrated in the exercise above, by clearing away excess mental clutter, and through meditation, which can be understood simply as thoughtless awareness. In meditation, we learn to watch our thoughts instead of getting hooked on them, and, consequently, we become the agent of our mental capacity instead of its victim.

But the very concept of "meditation" is likely surrounded by all kinds of pre-established thoughts that we might have. We are either drawn to the idea or repelled by it. We may think that to meditate we have to sit on a cushion in a lotus position and say "Om" in a very serious way for a certain period of time on a regular basis. But meditation isn't as complicated as we might want to make it. It is simply becoming conscious of wherever we are.

Awareness Exercise: Learning to Tune In

This exercise is designed as an introduction to meditation. It will give you an opportunity to experience the quieting of your mind. Sit where you are, but adjust your posture and uncross your legs and ankles so that you are in a comfortable yet well-balanced position with your feet flat on the floor, your spine as straight as possible, and one hand on each thigh (palms up or down, whichever feels more natural to you). You will need a few uninterrupted minutes.

1. Close your eyes and listen to all of the sounds that you can hear. Focus all of your attention on listening. If you catch yourself thinking about what you hear, just observe your thoughts and return to listening. If the space you are in is so quiet that there is not much

to listen to, then breathe deeply and focus on listening to your breath as it travels in and out. The exercise is to simply sit quietly with your eyes closed and listen to whatever sounds there may be.

2. After a few minutes, open your eyes and check in with yourself. Chances are that you feel a little bit peaceful. This is the result of quieting your mind. And in this quiet and neutral mind-space, it's possible to become aware of more than just the sounds in the room. We can learn to feel our internal state as well. Are we restless? Tired? Relaxed? Afraid?

3. Close your eyes again, maintain the same good sitting posture, and observe the way you feel on the inside. This is not about thinking about how you feel, but about tuning in to your internal state—your energy field, your nerves, and your gut. You are "taking a reading." And if you feel agitated, or out of sorts in any way, just breathe deeply, the whole length of your spine. Carry your breath like a wave down your vertebrae to the sacral bone, hold it there for a moment, and then release it like a wave back up your spine and out into space. Breathe deeply several times, and just focus on the traveling breath. Observe your energy change.

In this way, you can always restore yourself to neutrality, to an internal balance where you then have access to the flow of external energy as well. Internal awareness raises external awareness. We are then able to feel and sense the currents of things as they want to go, so that we needn't push against them. So much of our suffering comes from resisting life as it is. This state of being "in the flow" as described above, and hopefully experienced by you in the exercise, we will call spiritual fitness.

Learning to be simply observant of what is while remaining mentally neutral is a vital aspect of our good health and our well-being. Such a position allows for flexibility and curiosity and welcomes the unexpected. It sustains us and supports us as we explore the world and as we experience what life has to offer us on a daily basis. Another way to think of this is to have and maintain an open mind.

How We Feel about Ourselves and the Way We Eat

Our diet, as well as our thinking, is a direct reflection of our state of being. If we are not calm, balanced, and content, the way we eat will reveal our inner turmoil, as will the way we think. Our nourishment is our support. It promotes growth and sustains us over time. If we are reckless with our food choices by being overly permissive, drastically disciplined, or unconscious and unaware, that is a reflection of our internal state and our spiritual situation. So by better understanding how we feel on the inside, we can actually improve our relationship with food.

But it goes both ways, much like the chicken and the egg. The way we eat reflects our state of being, but our state of being is also reflected by the way we eat. They are both causes, and they are both effects. Sometimes, being hungry can instigate feelings of agitation and irritability, and sometimes, eating too much, or too much of the wrong thing, can make us feel sick, out-of-control, or upset. Food can either calm us or distress us, depending on what we eat and how we eat it. It's both a go-to place for the solution to our emotional imbalance and the potential cause of our internal unrest.

The goal must be to bring the internal and the external into alignment so that the one supports the other and we become able to maintain our best health and well-being. By simply raising our awareness to the food-emotion connection, we begin the process. It starts from wherever we are.

For my part, my relationship with food and with my body has been a long and harrowing journey. For many years, I was at war with portions, sweets, clothes, and the bathroom scale. Over time, I have come to understand that I was actually at war with myself. And I have had to change my habits and surrender to reality on multiple levels in order to feel safe and okay about who I am and how I look.

I used to eat out of boredom, compulsion, and emotional despair. I ate to celebrate and to numb my feelings. I always tried to maintain a perfect balance in order to have the right-size body, but I always missed the mark because I was never happy with myself the way I was. My thighs were too big and my stomach rolled over the top of my jeans when I sat down. I was relatively fit, and somewhat muscular, but I felt thick and fat—not feminine enough. And then I would have to eat in order to deal with my perceived lack of femininity, which contributed to greater thickness. It was a vicious cycle I was stuck in for years. My dysfunctional relationship with eating ruled me.

And yet, to look at me from the outside, I don't think it was at all obvious that I had "food issues." I was not particularly overweight by cultural standards, but on the inside, I felt horrible and huge. I understand now that it was a spiritual state as much as it was a physical one.

And then one year in late December, at the end of two months of holiday feasting and excess, I was sick to my soul of the food insanity and made an honest decision to address my issues. I stopped eating desserts entirely and almost passed out on day three from the change in my blood sugar. I had headaches and restlessness and felt like I was crawling out of my skin.

I wrote a daily journal to release emotional pressure and to keep track of my progress. I discovered that I habitually turned to food in general and sugar specifically when I was bored, tired, upset, overwhelmed, and afraid. Food was the place that I went for relief from the uncomfortable feeling of the moment, whatever that might be.

By monitoring myself over the course of a year, I realized that if I went too long without eating I became hostile and touchy. I also found that certain foods made me feel energized and jazzy and other foods made me feel grounded. I saw a connection between drinking coffee and irritability, between eating too much and feeling sickly full, and between not eating enough and feeling starved and weepy. It was quite a year of revelation.

I read books, talked to people, and shared my experience with others who understood and some who did not. I lost weight and gained weight. I did a weeklong steamed vegetable and sauna cleanse and briefly felt lean and beautiful. And after three months, I slowly reintroduced desserts into my life and observed that a bit of sugar made me crave more.

I learned about myself through this process. I learned that I had a belief system all around eating that was rooted in my childhood, and that I was programmed from a young age to be a dedicated member of the "clean plate club," no matter how much was on my plate. And I came to understand that this was true in relation to my life as well as to food. I wanted no loose ends and no unfinished business.

But over time, I learned that it was possible to be reasonable about what I ate and that I *could* eat anything, but that I didn't really want to. I learned that a few bites of something could actually be more satisfying than an endless and massive amount—in life as well as in my stomach—and I learned all about the insidious connection within me between nourishment and guilt.

I realized that for me, food had become a moral issue. I was "good" or "bad" depending on how successfully I was depriving myself of things that I wanted to eat and how much I weighed. I used food as reward and punishment both, which resulted in self-loathing and self-satisfaction over the same five pounds for decades. If I was up five I was miserable and felt fat and unattractive, and if I was down five I was happy. I came to realize that "weight" for me was an emotional and spiritual issue. Heavy or light was about my life as much as my body. My health with food was directly proportional to my health with everything.

As I became a better eater—not so much in terms of what I ate, but in how I ate—then my relationships, self-image, ability to be honest in other areas of my life, and feelings about my body all got better. And so did my courage to try new things. I became willing to speak up for myself and set boundaries.

In addition, I learned that many of us have the same kind of inner angst and turmoil over a few pounds, the latest diet, the second helping, and the lurching pendulum from permissiveness to deprivation. It's a torturous way to live, and it seems unstoppable. But we can stop. We can all find our way to make peace with food. Ultimately, it's an inside job, but it starts by changing external habits. I know that it works because I have done it. Although it may not be easy, it's entirely worth it. Life is simpler and supremely satisfying when we are not mentally obsessed with what we are eating or not eating and when we realize that we can be trusted to properly nourish ourselves.

Honesty Exercise: Where to Begin

Completing the checklist below will help identify issues surrounding your body image and the way you eat. You will need a pen or a pencil and a few minutes of quiet, uninterrupted time. Consider the statements below and put a check mark beside each one that rings "true." If the statement does not resonate, just leave it blank. Remember to be honest.

_____I am comfortable with my body just the way it is.

_____I am too tall.

_____I am too short.

_____I am too stocky.

_____I have body parts that I don't like.

_____I am overweight.

_____I am too thin.

_____I have a healthy, balanced diet and I rarely overeat.

_____I overeat on a regular basis.

_____I overeat desserts.

_____I overeat starches.

_____I overeat fried food.

_____I overeat fast food.

_____I rarely/sometimes/often (circle one)
eat to the point of sickness.

_____I sometimes feel guilty after eating.

_____I am a binge eater.

_____I am a late-night snacker.

_____I sometimes sneak food.

_____I rarely/sometimes/often (circle one) skip meals.

_____I do not drink enough water.

_____I drink too much coffee.

_____I drink too much soda.

_____I am always on a diet or thinking about dieting.

_____I feel good about myself when I am on
a diet and bad about myself when I am not.

_____I feel deprived when I am dieting.

_____I have a hard time sticking to a diet.

_____I flip-flop between being a disciplined
eater to being out of control.

_____I overregulate my food intake.

_____I have no discipline. I eat whatever I want.

_____I eat too fast.

_____I don't enjoy eating.

_____I do not stop eating when I am full.

_____I eat standing up or on the run.

_____I always clean my plate no matter what.

_____I eat when I'm bored.

_____I eat when I am stressed out or worried.

_____I can't trust myself with food.

_____Other: _____

Now, go back and write the number 1 beside the statement in this list that resonates the most strongly with you, and then do the same with numbers 2 and 3. Through this exercise, you have raised your awareness in some way regarding your habituated thoughts and behaviors surrounding food and your body. Consider this as information gathered, and keep it at the forefront of your mind as we proceed. We will refer back to this list in the next chapter.

What We Know: The Practical Facts

I am not a certified nutritionist and am not espousing any particular dietary path. But nonetheless, there are commonsense things that we all know in relation to food and our diets whether we admit them or not. We know that what we eat affects the way we feel. And we also know that what we eat can (and does) affect our overall health and our weight, which in turn affects our internal state, or "spiritual fitness." So there is a connection between what we choose to consume and the way we experience our lives and our bodies. This connection is a guarantee.

Another guarantee is that being overweight affects our mobility and, barring some medical condition or particular medication, it's possible for us to change the way our body feels and functions by eating less and moving more. We tend to overcomplicate this simple fact, though for the majority of us, it is a bottom line truth. If we burn more energy than we take in, our bodies have to use stored reserves to keep us going, and those stored reserves come in the form of fat, which is essentially unused, or blocked, energy. If we set this energy free by losing excess weight, then we are likely to feel better all over.

It is also the case that as adult individuals, we can eat anything we choose to eat. We have free will and a world full of grocery stores and restaurants to pick from. Anything that we do not eat, we choose not to eat. Sometimes the decision is pretty clear-cut—a shellfish allergy would compel us to avoid eating shrimp no matter what, because we don't want to go into anaphylactic shock and die. But the only thing that actually stands between ourselves and a shrimp cocktail is our clear decision not to eat it—our choice. We could eat it if we made the decision to do so, and we would suffer the consequences. The only thing stopping us is us, and our understanding of cause and effect. We choose not to eat shellfish because we don't want to get sick. The shellfish example demonstrates how easy it is to make a good choice when the stakes are high, but the consequences of most food choices are not as dramatic. Nonetheless, I would argue that the cause and effect relationships are often clearer than we think.

If we get acid indigestion every time after we eat pizza, then it's probably safe to say that pizza causes this effect on our system. Or if a basket of chips and salsa make us feel greasy, then that's the effect of chips and salsa. If we feel fat and guilty every time we eat a certain dessert, then fat and guilty are the effects of that dessert. The specific list of causes and effects are different for each individual, and it's your choice (and I would argue, your responsibility) to pay attention enough to be able to clearly know what your list is.

And we also know from experience that what we eat has a next-day effect as well. An overindulgence of rich foods and heavy sauces or an excess of sugar can give us a kind of food hangover the morning after. We might have a headache, or nausea, or feel clammy or crampy, or simply off our game. Certain foods disagree with us every time we eat them but we keep on eating them because for whatever reason we like the idea of them, or fail to connect the dots between the cause and effect. This can become particularly challenging if we have a delayed sensitivity.

The point is that the way specific foods act and react with our specific metabolisms is a topic that requires our self-honesty. Being realistic can give us a sense of power and control over the way that we feel, our health, and our happiness. When we eat this, we feel terrible. When we have that for dinner, we gain four pounds on the scale. When we prepare this food in this way we feel energized and healthy. When we eat too much of that food, we feel heavy and tired. Our bodies and our spirits will guide us to the best choices if we will only pay attention. (There is a "voice within" that speaks if we will listen: a point we address further in the next chapter.)

Something else that we all know about food whether we admit it or not is that fresh food or fresh-frozen food is better for us than processed food; the closer we can stay to the garden or the farm, the more "natural" the state of our food, the better. An apple is a better choice for our health and weight than an apple fritter. A piece of baked chicken is a better choice than chicken nuggets. A raw almond is better than one that is salted and roasted. And certain foods, although delicious in theory, have very little nutritional benefit at all, so eating them as anything more than an occasional tasty treat will not serve us in any kind of way. As a sweet they may satisfy our taste buds, but if we eat them as "food" we may be missing the point of what our "food" is supposed to be. This category might include frosted donuts, hot fudge sundaes and extreme desserts, a whole gamut of chips and packaged foods, nachos and cheese, and a litany of choices from fast food restaurant menus. The idea of them may be tempting, but the actual feeling we get from eating them is not completely satisfactory. Again, we know which foods are good for us in a healthy kind of way and which foods are less than beneficial. We know without a doubt.

More Practicality: Fats, Carbs, and Sugar

Continuing the discussion from a commonsense, layman's point of view, we can assert that "fats" in general get a bad rap in our culture. Some fats—like nuts, seeds, avocados, olive oil—are healthy and necessary, and if we eliminate too much of these from our diets, our bodies revolt and resist. The fat produced from these type of foods protects our internal organs, and if we are not providing it, the body will hold on to what it has in storage and not let go. If, however, we consume these healthy fats in balanced portions, our bodies engage in a trusting kind of give and take.

Carbohydrates, or "carbs," get a lot of negative press because in excess, more than other food groups, they contribute to unwanted weight gain. They are a ready source of body energy. Brown rice, a baked potato, or a tangerine are healthy carbohydrate choices. Within a reasonable number of hours after eating these types of foods, our body can use them to move muscles and to energize physical labor. They act like gas in a car. They power the engine.

But if we do not burn carbohydrates through physical motion, our bodies transform them into fat for backup energy at some point in the future. Consequently, we develop excess fat stores when we overeat carbohydrates. The key is to appropriately balance our complex carbohydrate intake with our physical output if we want to maintain a certain weight. If we want to lose weight and lose fat, then we need to have a higher energy output than we do carbohydrate intake.

It works like this: if we need energy to get moving or to stay moving, but don't have carbs ready and available to use, then our body will draw upon fat stores and transform the fat into energy, which is exactly what we want to have happen if we want to shrink our size. If we need to gain weight, eating complex carbohydrates like whole grains, beans, and other root vegetables is a good place to begin.

The biggest problem for many of us has to do with refined carbohydrates: candy bars, potato chips, crackers, pretzels, white bread, soda and energy drinks, many fruit juices, and anything made with white or all-purpose flour. These are the "less than beneficial" food family described in the section above. Processed and often loaded down with sugar, these foods set a physical craving in motion that makes us want more of them. I have found that I cannot consume refined carbohydrates except in minimal portions if I want to relate in a healthy way to the food I eat, and I believe that this is true for most of us. Refined carbohydrates and sugar are the primary saboteurs of a lean and healthy body.

Sugar, as well as being sweet and tasty, is addictive. It does not have any nutritional benefit, and it takes our whole energy system on a wild ride every time we eat it, especially in excess. Consider for a moment what a piece of cake or a candy bar will do to a young child. In adults it may be less obvious, but it does the same thing.

Eating sweets spikes our blood sugar to an abnormally high level, which then triggers our body to release insulin in order to regulate the system. Too much sugar equals too much insulin, which then crashes our blood sugar, depleting us of energy. And then we tend to turn right back to sugar again because we crave the initial "high" that we experienced. Eating sugar makes us crave more sugar. This is how an addictive cycle begins. And the cycle can continue ad infinitum.

It's worth mentioning that sugar highs do burn energy, a fact that we can readily observe in children who are "bouncing off the walls" after eating too much of it, but burning energy this way is not efficient. The sugar that remains in the system once our insulin rush has come to lower the blood levels is stored, for future use, as fat.

So our best bet is to eat sugar in small bits, as a true-to-form, once-in-a-while "treat," eat the bulk of our healthy carbs early in the day so that we have the ready ability to burn them as we move about through our activities, and eat minimal carbs for dinner. And if we want to lose weight, we should eat as little sugar and as few carbs as possible at all times, while continuing to eat a reasonable amount of healthy fats and drink plenty of water.

We have to be a bit cautious when it comes to fruit because fruits are carbs—good carbs, but carbs, nonetheless—and fruit is also high in sugar, which is natural sugar, but sugar nonetheless, and still affects the blood and insulin levels. To maintain a lean and healthy body, it has been my experience that lean protein, lots of veggies, and a small portion of healthy fat, with occasional complex carbohydrates, and even-more-occasional sweets, makes for the ultimate diet.

Even if we exercise regularly, this balanced diet makes sense. While it's true that athletes require more carbs than average because of their intense physical demands and energetic output, most of us, even if we're fit, do not fall into this category. Much as we may want it to be the case, or want to talk ourselves into it, "carb loading" is not necessary for an average workout at the gym.

All of the above is general information based on my opinion and my understanding of nutrition; it does not represent absolute truth. It is what I have learned, experienced, and chosen to share with you to be helpful. But ultimately, I direct you back to yourselves. If you disagree strongly with anything that I have said, I encourage you to honor yourself. Diet and dietary opinion is a personal matter, and we all have to discover the path that is the right one for us. Some of us are all about raw foods, and some of us are all about macrobiotics; some are low-carb, some are all-fruit, some are paleo, and some are pescatarians. The point, and the purpose, is to find what works for you. If you feel great eating what you're eating—keep eating it. But if you don't feel great, then perhaps the guidelines and suggestions above might be helpful as you journey forth. That is my hope.

Understanding Hunger and the Importance of Accountability

Also in my experience, and as a general rule, I have come to understand that every time we feel hungry, we assume that food will satisfy us. But sometimes, it doesn't. Sometimes, we are hungry for something other than food; something deeper, or something different. We are beings with a whole host of sensual and spiritual needs. Perhaps when we feel hungry we are actually hungry for beauty, or light. Maybe our cramped, dark office and endless rows of computers and closed doors have depressed us, and we need to get out in the sun for a bit and see trees and people and the earth.

Or maybe we are hungry for the scent of something delicate and delicious—the aroma of rain if it's been parched and hot, or the smells of the body and physical closeness, or wood smoke on a winter day. Maybe we're hungry for deep breaths of fresh air, the feeling of soft cotton, a provocative movie, or a good book. Or maybe we are dehydrated and in need of water.

Our appetites are vast, and we intuitively seek balance. If we have been alone too long, we hunger for the noise and energy of a crowd. We hunger for touch, for comfort, for intellectual stimulation, for sleep. We hunger for appreciation. We hunger for love. We hunger for approval, mastery, physical fitness, and spiritual insight. We hunger for a whole world of sensual and emotional satisfaction, and it's up to us to be able to identify what we're actually hungry for at any given time, because a piece of buttered bread will not satisfy our hunger for light or beauty or conversation.

If we try to fill our hunger with food and food is not what we're hungry for, then no amount of food will fill us up. But this doesn't stop us, because there is a certain comfort in the numbing effect of chewing, swallowing, and filling our stomachs to the brim. But at the end of it all, when we are sick from eating too much, we are as lonely as we were before, or as disappointed, or as bored. The only difference is that we have given ourselves something to distract us from reality. And that satisfaction is limited at best.

We cannot expect to live in healthy balance with food if we are unwilling to learn the ongoing art of self-honesty and the regular practice of tuning in to our internal selves. Our relationship to what we eat does not exist in a vacuum. Everything depends upon it and it depends upon everything else: the way we think, the way we feel, the things we long for, and all of our hopes and fears. Perhaps we are deficient in a certain vitamin or mineral, or our hormones are out of whack, and we need a blood test to determine what's going on. Honestly admitting that something is amiss begins the journey to its proper correction.

If we are angry or hurt, the agitation we feel will not be eliminated by a piece of chocolate cake smothered in whipped cream. That may suppress the upset feelings but it will not release them. We have to learn how to process our lives and the things that happen to us, and we have to know and ask for what we need— what we really need, not to escape or pretend but to deal with the reality of our lives.

Maybe that doesn't sound like much fun. Maybe the chocolate cake seems like the better option right now, but it won't be in the long run. Whether we stuff ourselves with food out of anxiety, boredom, or whatever, in the end, we have to face the truth of our life. That's the spiritual reality. We may be able to put off our uncomfortable feelings and heartaches for a while in an overflowing bowl of ice cream or a pasta fest, but we cannot send them packing. We can pretend not to see them. We can throw food at them for weeks, but no matter our antics, they wait for us. They wait for us for as long as it takes. And we have to deal with them eventually.

So why not deal with them as they come up? When we feel hungry let's learn to understand the difference between lunchtime and hurt feelings. One is an emptiness in the stomach and the other is an emptiness in the soul. To determine which is which, we can examine changes in our behavior.

If we find ourselves compulsively craving sweets or other delicacies in a manner that is unusual for us, or if we cannot eat enough to fill us up, then something deeper is likely going on. But how do we figure out what it is? And how do we fix it? And how do we *not* eat when everything inside of us wants to consume whatever we can reach?

It's honesty first and foremost, and the ability to pause long enough before gorging to look within, to identify that something emotional and unidentified is, in fact, going on, and then to ask ourselves why? That's the deeper layer. And sometimes it takes a pretty sincere effort to trace ourselves back to the incident that may have disrupted our lives. It could be rooted in something from our past, or some anxiety about the future, or something someone said or did. We have to learn ourselves. That's the goal.

It's easy to face facts in our minds, but in doing so, we may often miss important details that make all the difference in the end. To keep track of everything we eat everyday is asking an awful lot of ourselves and is probably unrealistic over any length of time. But to keep track of what we eat and how it makes us feel for a few days, a week, or as long as it's useful, is doable and reasonable. And what it may teach us is well worth the effort. It's easy to convince ourselves that we didn't eat much, or that we feel great after wolfing down a huge dessert. But if we have to check in with ourselves and actually articulate exactly what we did eat—and exactly how we do feel—then we may learn something.

Honesty Exercise:
What We Are Actually Eating, and Why?

Keeping a food log, as this exercise suggests, will make you accountable for what you eat. You will need your journal or a downloaded app for your smartphone that allows you to track your food consumption. The app, if that's the route you go, will need to allow you to make comments. I happen to be a great believer in the power of writing things down. The process of handwriting engages the senses in such a way that the very act of it can be transformative, so I heartily suggest the use of your journal over a cell phone. But the exact method is secondary to the willingness, so there's no need to get hung up on it.

The point, and the exercise, is to track your food consumption for at least a few days, preferably a week or more, leaving out nothing, and incorporating commentary on how you feel both before and after you eat. Check in with yourself and take note of any sensations at any time—irritability, boredom, restlessness, self-satisfaction, or whatever you may feel. You may need to store your feelings and the details of your intake in memory until you have a chance to put them down, but the idea is to consistently track them as many times a day as you need to.

EXAMPLE: DAY ONE: SUNDAY

6:00 am: I woke up feeling calm and centered, had a glass of water with lemon, took a short walk, and then sat down at my computer.

7:00 am: Agitated and nervous-feeling—almost fearful. Had a cup of tea, two pieces of toast, a few walnuts, and two dried figs. I ate all of this unconsciously while continuing to work at the computer, and drank the tea fast, almost compulsively. I felt better and more grounded, but had no sense of having appreciated the meal.

8:30 am: Agitated again—and hungry-feeling. Drank a glass of water and had another cup of tea. I noticed that I wasn't breathing deeply so I took a few deep breaths, which helped; started to drink the tea fast again, but I caught myself and made a conscious effort to slow down.

9:30 am: Went outside—beautiful day. Felt good, hopeful, happy. Had another glass of water sitting on the porch.

10:00 am: Brunch at a local restaurant with my husband. Drank three cups of coffee and ate two poached eggs and rye toast, a pancake with butter (no syrup)—and a few bites of bacon. I felt overfull and tired after—irritable, even a little depressed. Worked outside in the garden for a few hours when we got home and felt better.

2:00 pm: Late lunch—a carrot, some leftover lamb from dinner last night, and half of a small sliced tomato from the garden. I was aware of having to really chew the carrot, so that slowed me down, and I paid attention while I was chewing the lamb as well. I usually eat way faster than my husband and I kept pace with him for a change, which felt good, as did the meal.

4:30 pm: A glass of water. Trying to stave off rising hungry feelings and make it until dinner without eating…

5:40 pm: Hungry! A bit edgy; 45 minutes to dinner; feeling amped and a bit excitable, don't want to snack…

5:45 pm: Couldn't stand it—had a small dried fig and a few almonds—felt immediately better.

6:30 pm: Sat down for dinner—ate a grilled chicken thigh, a mini baked sweet potato from our garden (the first of the year and the first I've ever grown—it was delicious!) and a serving of sautéed spinach. I was more mindful about eating more slowly than usual, but I still beat my husband. I felt like I could eat more when I was finished, but I didn't. We sat and talked, and I realized as we sat that I was perfectly satisfied.

After dinner, I had a cup of ginger tea and three Maria cookie/crackers for dessert—ate at my computer—drank the tea too fast. Felt tired, a little fuzzy mentally, and the Sunday night back-to-work-in-the-morning feeling setting heavily in.

Through the process of doing this exercise for even one day, we are returned to the food-mood connection as articulated earlier in the chapter. The way we eat reflects our state of being, but our state of being is also reflected by the way we eat. So now that we have all of these facts, all of this information, personal honesty, and awareness, what now? How on earth are we supposed to change?

Believing We're Worth It

It starts by believing that change is possible. This is a very important point. Belief is a strange and powerful transformational tool; without it, we are unlikely to sustain any changes that we might make. We have to believe that we are worth the effort. If spiritual fitness, good health, and well-being are our goals, they can become our reality, but we have to be willing to believe in the feasibility of the long-term process.

And perhaps, our belief will grow as we experience success making small changes in our habits, and then grow stronger still as we change further. But initially, we have to at least want something better than what we have, and be willing to believe that we can have it. Affirmations are a useful tool to help us to do that.

Willingness Exercise: Affirmations to Create Momentum

By consistently repeating an affirmation to yourself, you can effectively program your mind to cooperate with your physical and spiritual goals. You will need a pen or a pencil and a few quiet, uninterrupted moments. Underline an affirmation from the list below that feels "right" to you, or create one of your own beginning with the statement "I am willing…" or "I believe…" Keep it as simple as possible.

+ I am willing to love my body and feed it with care.

+ I am willing to eat mindfully.

+ I am willing to positively change the way that I think about food and about my body.

+ I am willing to eat a healthy amount for my body's needs.

+ I am willing to take good care of myself.

+ Other: I am willing to _____

+ I believe I can feel good about my body and my diet.

+ I believe that positive change is possible for me.

+ I believe that I can enjoy healthy eating.

+ I believe that I can successfully change my food habits, adjust or maintain my weight according to what is most healthy for my body, and feel great!

+ I believe that I can eat what I love
  and love my body at the same time.

+ Other: I believe _____

Use whichever affirmation you choose. Say it out loud or quietly to yourself every morning when you wake up and every evening before you go to sleep, and any other time throughout the day when it occurs to you. This process helps get the wheel of change turning steadily and keeps it moving forward.

One of the ways we set ourselves up for failure in changing our habits is to want too much change too quickly and to demand so much of ourselves that we cannot possibly maintain our endurance. This is the case with so many radical diets and with exercise programs that begin on January first. They are impractical for the long haul. We need to keep it simple and grow our willingness slowly over time. The affirmation that we choose can help us to do that, and prepares us for the next step.

CHAPTER TWO

· ·

Turning Honesty
into Health as a Habit

"One half of knowing what you want is
knowing what you must give up to get it."
—Sidney Howard

At old-fashioned mills, the grinding wheel operates by the power of water falling. Momentum builds over time, making it turn faster and faster, and as long as the water falls, the wheel turns. If the water stops for some reason, the wheel keeps turning for a period of time because, as Newton stated, "a force in motion tends to stay in motion." The only way to stop it quickly is to engage some kind of counter-force. Much like placing a finger on a spinning top or coin, a sudden, jarring cross-friction is the only thing that can arrest the movement.

Our habits of thought and self-talk, our behaviors, desires, fears, and compulsions are like the water on the wheel. They will continue to turn us round and round in cycles forever unless we use a certain power and counterforce to stop the momentum. That counterforce is our intention, our willingness, and our belief that things in our lives can be better than they are and that we can feel better than we currently feel.

Food habits are particularly tricky in this regard. It's not like cigarettes or alcohol where we can just quit cold turkey. We cannot stop eating. But what we can do is stop the specific eating habit that is causing us the most trouble. If we are late-night snackers, then we can STOP late-night snacking. If we are fast food fanatics, then we can STOP eating fast food, maybe not forever, but at least at the beginning. If yo-yo dieting is creating dysfunction in our lives then we can STOP yo-yo dieting. From everything I know and have experienced, it's a lost cause to believe we can somehow "modify" out-of-control behavior. We may be able to eventually, but at first we have to STOP the momentum. We have to engage the powerful counterforce. If we only slow down the dripping water, the wheel is still pulling us around and around.

Using the results from the "Where to Begin" exercise from the last chapter (pages 28–31), and any relevant findings to date from your food journal, determine your biggest source of food dysfunction—the thing regarding your eating habits that causes you more angst and discomfort than anything else—and make the decision to STOP doing it. And then, using the affirmation that you chose or created and believing that change is possible, simply STOP, and commit to staying stopped. That's more than enough. Making this kind of dramatic change is generally excruciating, especially for the first week or so. We are habituated to our routine. We plop in front of the television with our bowl of ice cream. So if we don't have it, we feel at a loss. That is to be expected. Change is not easy.

I believe that all of our dysfunctional food habits are like the turning waterwheel, and if we want to stop them, we have to STOP. But it's the biggest and baddest one first—the one that makes us cringe every time we think of it. We have to prioritize which habits to change. Like putting a tourniquet on an open wound to control the bleeding, the most urgent need has to be addressed first, and once that's under control, then the additional damage can be assessed.

The body will rebel and so will our psyche. Our strong desire and physical urge is to return to the equilibrium that we know. If we are in the habit of treating ourselves to a handful of cookies every night after dinner, there is a vacancy in our world—an electrical socket that has been unplugged. And it's far easier to plug something else in than to leave the socket empty. In fact, it's necessary if we want to succeed. We have to reprogram our minds and our bodies to a new routine of behavior to fill the gap and the space and the time. Maybe something completely different, like taking a moonlight walk around the block or drinking herbal tea could work for us. Or maybe playing with a straw, chewing gum, or busying our hands with a project. These suggestions may seem like a far cry from our favorite cookies, but they will fill the void and distract us.

Bringing about lasting change is a long process, not a quick fix, and it necessarily starts with a certain amount of discomfort. Getting through a whole week with a new habit is hard to do. The second week is easier, and the third week easier still. And if we can stick with it, after only a few months, we hardly even miss the old pattern. This is the path and the way to enlightened living. It takes initial discomfort, but it does get easier over time.

It's like turning an enormous cruise ship. It's so big that it turns by only slight angles at a time and hardly even seems to be moving at all, and yet, it is moving and it does turn, and eventually it is heading straight in an entirely new direction. We are like that cruise ship. We have to change by degree.

Diets often fail before they begin because they are set up as a short-term solution to a set of well-established lifetime habits. When they are over, the old patterns return, and the weight that has been lost is recovered again. Diets can turn a day-sailor or a kayak, but not a cruise ship.

If we want peace with food and don't have it, then we need a long-term sustainable solution, and not a quick fix. But in order to achieve that, we have to be willing to experience discomfort in our lives. As Antoine de Saint-Exupery said in *The Little Prince*, "(We) must be willing to endure the presence of a few caterpillars if (we) wish to become acquainted with the butterflies."

So our first mindful action is to STOP the wheel of greatest dysfunction and then settle in for however long it takes to adapt, relatively speaking, to the new routine: probably at least a few weeks, and at most, if we're vigilant, a few months. We may continue to have moments of discomfort that last longer than that, but they will come less and less often, and with ever less intensity as we begin to realize that we can survive, and actually be okay, without habitually indulging in our daily cookies, fast food stop, or Friday night chip-and-dip fest.

We can be okay without overeating at every meal, without skipping meals, without dieting or stringently restricting ourselves at every turn, and without cleaning our plate. We can be better than okay. We can learn to trust ourselves and allow for pleasure in the process. And as we shift away from our number-one dysfunctional habit in relation to food, we can look at what remains with courage and even a bit of confidence.

Whatever the second-biggest problem is for us, that's the one to deal with second and in the same fashion (refer again to the "Where to Begin" exercise results and your food journaling).

The answer to our food issues is not the perfect four-week diet plan, a pill, or a session of hypnosis, but ongoing self-honesty and the continued willingness to face the real truth about ourselves and make appropriate changes where they are called for.

It does need to be said here that anorexia, bulimia, morbid obesity, and other medical and psychological conditions that directly impact our food intake and our weight may require outside help to work through. And if any of these happen to be your condition, please be honest about that and get the help you need.

But for most of us, we have garden-variety food dysfunction. We starve ourselves to fit into clothes that we bought a size too small, and then reward ourselves with excessive overindulgence, which leaves us with residual guilt. We sway all over the map and wonder why we never feel steady. We can get steady. It is within our power to do so.

Planning Carefully

From our discussion in the last chapter and our journaling efforts, hopefully we are learning to understand the difference between emotional and physical hunger. Once we "get it," then it's important to honor our physical hunger in certain and particular ways. If we grab at anything available and gulp it down half-consciously while continuing to work, drive, or carry on other business, we are missing an important opportunity for pleasure and sustenance in our lives. We are missing out on the spiritual satisfaction of mindful eating.

We eat regularly; that is a fact of being alive. We require meals, snacks, and water, and if we pretend that we can skip these things, we are fooling ourselves. Some of us can eat less than others. Some of us require only two meals a day, or five small meals, but we all need to eat something at certain intervals as we go about living our lives. Knowing this, it is incredible to me how easily we tend to blow this fact off.

We head out into the world for a day of activity and don't bother to consider in advance how we are going to address our hunger needs. We don't carry snacks or water, don't plan lunch, and cavalierly figure that we will simply "grab something" when we get hungry. But what if we're not close to anything healthy when we get hungry? Or not close to anything period?

One thing I have learned about myself is that when I go too long without eating, I become edgy and irritable and crawly inside my skin. I get almost desperate-feeling. And I have witnessed the same effect in others to greater or lesser degrees. This is one obvious way that food intake and moods are directly related. So when we skip eating because there's nothing convenient to "grab," our sense of well-being deteriorates steadily the longer we hold out, and rather than feeling thin and successful, we feel hostile, and we unknowingly set in motion what I will call the "starvation syndrome." We allow ourselves to become so hungry that when we finally do have the opportunity to eat, we do so in a kind of frenzy. We eat fast and furiously and take big bites, and we cannot get our fill until we are overstuffed. And then we likely feel frustrated because we ended up eating more than we intended to, or than we needed. There is nothing mindful or pleasurable in this kind of behavior.

The potential for this unfortunate chain of events, which I'm quite sure has happened to all of us at one time or another, is easily avoided with a little bit of forethought. Considering our day in advance can save us hours of angst. Again, though, we have to get honest—especially if we are regularly on a diet and habitually tell ourselves that we will simply skip lunch. Even if it never quite pans out that way, we continue to trust in our willpower over our nature. And while it's possible to not eat out of sheer determination, there is a price to pay for that choice, and it generally backfires on us in the end. We skip lunch and then aggressively overeat at dinner.

So it's a crucial step to get truthful with ourselves about the fact that we do, in fact, get hungry at regular intervals, and we do, in fact, need to eat whether we're on a diet or not, working all day or not, shopping or not, taking care of small children, taking care of aging parents, on vacation, visiting friends, or all of the above or none of the above. No matter what, we need to eat.

So, that being the case even if we may not want it to be, then it's worth spending a few minutes to consider where we might be in our day when we are likely to get hungry, and to get in the habit of carrying contingency supplies with us. Appropriate preparation may be one of the most important factors in our dietary success. Let's learn to pack a healthy lunch, to have snacks available, to carry water bottles, and to never have to experience that state of urgent, desperate hunger that drives us to the fast food location down the block, to the vending machine, or to the plate of cookies in the break room. And though we object to this simple idea on so many levels—we don't have time, we're not that organized, or whatever our excuse might be—we can learn how to be prepared and experience a whole new level of self-confidence and control in our lives. Taking care of ourselves in this way is spirituality in action.

Our preparation begins at the store and in our pantries and refrigerators. What we buy and what we keep around the house makes a difference. We have to be honest here as well. We can err on the side of not having enough to satisfy us as well as having too much that is rich and fatty and junky. So often, with the best of intentions, we buy masses of vegetables that we think will be good for us, or nothing but lettuce, and it all ends up rotting in the drawer as we scour our shelves for something with more substance. We have to learn to honor the need for balance in our lives if we want to achieve a state of emotional balance, good health, and well-being.

We need food variety in the course of each day. We need complex carbohydrates, vegetables, protein, and a bit of healthy fat, or some other combination of options that satisfies us and makes us feel great. This is a personal journey and we have to do what suits us best. Arguably, we may even need a taste of sweetness included in our daily fare, if we have a sweet tooth, in order to bypass feelings of deprivation. What we eat is our choice and we can choose what we like. And we may think that we want nothing but sweets or nothing but salad, but neither of those is realistic. To feel its best, our body craves equilibrium. External balance begets internal balance. The effects of our healthy or poor choices travel both ways.

We have a tendency to set ourselves up in opposition to our flesh and bones as if they are the enemy and somehow keep us from being able to indulge in what we think we want. And yet, what we really want, if we're honest, is what makes us feel the best, and our bodies are on board here. But they are cooperative no matter how dysfunctional we are. They go along and reflect our choices perfectly. The error is not in our bodies, but in us. If we believe that we should be able to eat nothing but processed food, sugar, and whatever is most readily available and still have an exquisite figure and good health to show for it, perhaps we are the enemy of our bodies, and not the other way around.

If we want a lean, energized body, then we need to eat lean, energizing foods. "We are what we eat" is a true statement. And we eat better if we consider our options in advance and plan ahead when our options are limited. One way to do this is to prepare on-the-road meals for ourselves—to pack breakfast, or lunch, or whatever meal we will miss at home. There is comfort in knowing that when we are hungry, wherever we may be, we have something uniquely delicious prepared just for us waiting and ready in our cooler or the company fridge or wherever. It gives us roots of sorts in our day, and anchors us in healthy goodness.

And it needn't be difficult or complex: a small piece of baked chicken or salmon in a Tupperware dish, hard-boiled eggs, spinach leaves, leftover vegetables from dinner the night before, carrot sticks, Wasa crackers, nuts, cheese, an apple, spaghetti squash with fresh ginger, whatever our imagination can think of and our body likes. Having satisfying meals such as these prepared in advance saves us time and angst.

It is hard, however, and maybe even impossible, to add one more thing to our already full morning routines, so it's much easier on us and everyone around us if we pack our lunch the night before, or our breakfast for the next day, or snacks, or whatever it is.

Being Prepared at Home

Preparing meals at home requires forethought as well. Frozen dinners, cans of soup, prepackaged meals, deli meats, macaroni and cheese, and options along these lines may be easy, but they may not be our best choice if we want to feel great. We need to remember that the closer we stay to the farm and the fresher our food, the better it is for us and the better we will feel.

That being said, we can purchase about a week's worth of meals at a time. It's helpful to make a list and to know what we are planning to prepare in advance. This may seem overwhelming.

How on earth do we know on Sunday what we want to eat for dinner on Wednesday? Or lunch on Friday?

If we take the time to properly take stock of our tastes, then we know what we like and what we don't like, what suits us and what does not. And chances are, we eat basically the same things in a rotating fashion anyway, so it's not nearly as complicated as we think. For me, the basics are the most satisfying: basic proteins and basic vegetables and easy on the starch. A couple of sample weekday dinners in my household might look something like this: grilled chicken, steamed asparagus, and sliced tomatoes; or, baked salmon, sautéed spinach, and steamed kale; or, poor man's steak (marinated chuck roast on the grill), a small baked red potato, and steamed broccoli. But we all have different preferences.

The point is to consider our menu in advance. If we know that we are planning to have a particular meal for dinner, then we can anticipate it throughout the day and develop an appetite for it. I find this far more fulfilling than being like a pinball and not knowing what I am doing—whether I am going out or staying in and what I am going to eat. Meal planning in a reckless, last-minute kind of way on a daily basis can be stressful, and unnecessarily so. Making our dinner choices in advance anchors us in the same way our packed lunch does at work. At least, this has been my experience.

Since so much of our discomfort in life comes from uncertainty—from all of the things that we can't control and that can't be controlled—in areas where we do have the control, why not assert it? It makes for a much calmer daily ride. This is practical, spiritual practice. It doesn't have to be esoteric. Having what we need for five or six well-balanced days of meals removes an incredible amount of strain from the effort of life. We simply prepare the food in advance, and delight in the eating of it later.

This brings up another important point: the preparation of food. It makes a difference whether it is made with love and good humor, or whether it is thrown together with haste and irritability. Cooking with care, like planning with care, is spiritual practice.

One Sunday, my husband and I compulsively decided that we wanted to roast a turkey. It seemed like just the thing to do. But we couldn't find a fresh one locally, so we bought one frozen and set about trying to thaw it in an abbreviated fashion. We soaked it in hot water and ran it under the faucet, but this achieved limited success, so we ended up poking at it and prodding it and pulling at the wings and the bag of gizzards and trying to force it to thaw by all of our power and muscle. And eventually, we did get it soft enough to cook.

Hours later, when we sat down to eat it, it was the roughest, toughest turkey either of us had ever tasted. It had taken on all of the aggression that we had turned on it. I learned then without a doubt what I had always heard and believed; that the energy we bring to preparing food really does matter and that it makes a difference whether we cook with frustration or love.

I have been to restaurants and tasted the love that the chef has invested in the preparation of my food, and I have equally tasted the rush and the frenzy of other chefs. And I have enjoyed my own meals in varying degrees depending on the state of mind that I brought to the kitchen on that particular day or evening.

Eating Mindfully

If we are conscious, or lucky, and our meal has been prepared with care, then the next place to direct our awareness is on the energy that we bring to the eating itself. Do we wolf it down or take small bites and savor it? If we consistently eat in a rush, then I would be willing to bet that we are living in a rush. The way we eat reflects the way we live and vice versa. But what's our hurry? Why can't we slow down? And what are we missing if we don't? Arguably, perhaps, we are missing the whole point, which is to practice the art of good habits and, consequently, experience the benefits of good living.

Eating mindfully will change the way that we experience food, and potentially the way that we experience life as well. Mindfulness as a way-of-living concept is popular currently, and rather a "buzzword," but the truth is that it's been around for centuries. It originated in the East and is grounded fundamentally in Buddhism, but its application is unlimited across time and across cultures.

But what does it really mean? To be mindful? To eat mindfully? First and foremost, it means that we slow down and pay attention. It means that we say thank you before we begin and that we chew with awareness and appreciation, that we notice textures and flavors and subtleties of taste, and that we eat sitting down and pause briefly in between bites.

We miss so much enjoyment by rushing through our meals. We eat to fill a hole, to amp us up, to check off a box. We eat without care. We eat without notice. And then we leave the table hungry still. We miss the pleasure almost every time, except on special occasions, and even then we tend to make the experience more about the people and our outfits and hair than the delicacy of the food itself.

Eating mindfully means that we indulge in the goodness of good food, that we feel our bodies receive what we give them, and that we hear the response of our stomachs and inner energies to the meals we consume. It also means that we know what is soothing to us and what is not, and when we are satisfied and have had enough.

Our cultural habit of grab-and-go deprives us of sensational and spiritual delight that is meant for us on a regular basis. Our eating is meant to be restorative. It's meant to be a break and a rejuvenation, a pleasure and a soulful satisfaction. And we miss it by simply not paying attention. I would be willing to bet that we miss it nine times out of ten.

But it doesn't have to be that way. Slowing down doesn't have to be complicated, and it can change everything about our experience in a positive direction. When we slow down, one bite can encompass a world. When we slow down, our food has the potential to excite our tongues and teeth and taste buds, and awaken us from the inside out.

Any guide to good health will tell us that for optimal digestion and proper consumption, we should be chewing each bite of food twenty to thirty times. I challenge us all to do that—for only a few bites each day. That will slow us down. And likely make us eat less, and appreciate the intricacies of food flavor more. It is an interesting experiment. And it may not be realistic to chew every bite for that long in our world of fast-paced nonstop action and demand, but if we can shift even slightly in that direction, we can experience a corresponding shift of energy within.

And as within so without. If we can learn to savor our meals, we may learn to savor our experiences and the people we encounter and our feelings and our lives. In this way, our food may, in fact, be a gateway to enlightenment.

Awareness Exercise: Eating Mindfully Meditation

By eating slowly and consciously and by bringing your full awareness to the act of chewing, and the sensation of tasting, you will come to experience food in a complete and satisfying way. You will need a place to sit and a table, a healthy snack of your choosing, and a few moments of quiet, uninterrupted time.

1. Carefully prepare your snack on a small plate and make it look appealing.

2. Set a place for yourself at a table, clear of clutter, and sit down with your prepared plate.

3. Take a moment to appreciate what you are about to eat. Observe the color, the texture, the scent, and the presentation.

4. Slowly, and consciously, take a small bite. Close your eyes and tune all of your attention to chewing and tasting and observing. Chew at least twenty-five times before you swallow.

5. Take a second bite and keep your eyes open. Look around the room as you are chewing and focus on whatever captures your attention. Eat as you usually do, without all the ceremony of bite number one.

6. Take another slow and conscious bite like you did before with your eyes closed. Pay attention to chewing and tasting and the texture of the food in your mouth. And once again, chew at least twenty-five times before you swallow.

7. As you finish your snack, experiment with the two approaches and notice the differences between them. Which is more satisfying? Why?

By simply raising your awareness and paying attention to the process of chewing and tasting and swallowing, you can transform the simple act of having a snack into a sensual delight. This is the art of mindful eating, and the gateway to enlightenment of which we spoke.

The Voice that Tells Us When

Also available to us as a path to potential enlightenment is a voice within that speaks to us with certainty and clarity. It is not loud, not aggressive, and consequently, easy to ignore. But it is accurate, and it guides us perfectly if we will only listen.

This voice, among other things, tells us what we need, what we should and should not do, and when we have had enough to eat. Every time we sit down to a meal, it registers our appropriate finishing point. There is a definitive satiation message that we receive. But most of us are not in the habit of listening to it. We are, on the other hand, in the habit of drowning it out in conversation, music, distraction, more food—whatever is most readily available. What we rarely do is stop eating and push our plate away.

And yet, if we were able to register the message and act upon it, we would be our ideal weight. Our body knows exactly what it wants and needs for nourishment, and does not have a desire to overeat. Nonetheless, we tend to force extras upon it every day in the form of whatever appeals to our other senses, our psyches, and our emotional upheavals: pretty presentations of sweet treats, decadent plates of overflowing pasta, extra-large portions of anything and everything, bite-sized hors d'oeuvres, warm bread, creamy dips …

The advertising market is selling to everything in us that is in the habit of ignoring our inner voice. It appeals to our longings and our desire for guilt-free indulgence. We are promised satisfaction, great taste, and emotional security for a penny and a song. But it's all fantasy. It's improbable at best that the skinny model in the advertisement is really enjoying the special low-fat ice cream topped with chocolate. She is more likely half-starved and eating teeny-tiny portions, only just enough to survive. Or she might not be real at all. She might be a photoshopped manipulation.

Nonetheless, we somehow think that we can look like the picture if we eat the dessert. We deceive ourselves willingly and with enthusiasm. We don't listen to our inner guide and the still, small voice within that knows better and knows the truth.

We can learn to at least hear the voice, even if we are not yet ready to listen to it. We can take note when it speaks up. There it is, telling us we have had enough as we plunge forward with lustful abandon. There it is, saying not to eat the second helping of nachos, warning against the greasy fried chicken wings, the whole helping of cake and ice cream, the spicy peppers and onions.

We may recall its warnings later as we sit miserably with indigestion and a bloated stomach. "I knew I shouldn't have eaten that," we bemoan, but it is too late. Let's learn to listen right when the message comes in and trust that it is there for a reason and comes bearing glad tidings for us and not to sabotage our good time.

We fundamentally don't trust ourselves, that's the problem. We trust everything else before we will pay attention to what we instinctively know. We trust advertisers, friends, hearsay, the media; we trust whatever we hear and see and want to believe. The one thing we do not trust is the one thing that can change our life, simplify everything, and improve the quality of our every minute experience. It's the voice within. It's wise and knows what's best. Let's learn to hear it, to listen to it, and to follow its lead.

Awareness Exercise:
Learning to Listen to the Voice Within

By paying attention, as suggested in this exercise, you can learn to hear and eventually listen to the voice within. Making a habit of this will improve your overall well-being. The exercise requires your cooperation and willingness.

1. Bring a bit of extra awareness and an open mind to your next meal, and after you've eaten for a bit, see if you can hear the internal voice that tells you when you have had enough. Don't overthink it, and don't worry if you don't hear it.

2. Bring awareness to the next meal, and listen for the voice again.

3. When you do hear the voice, and you will eventually, observe your reaction to it. Do

you stop eating as it suggests? Or do you completely ignore it, or otherwise blow it off?

4. Keep listening for the voice in an ongoing way, and when you hear it, do what it suggests. This is easier said than done, but doing it can transform your entire relationship to food, to life, and to happiness and fulfillment in general, so it's well worth the effort.

By learning to hear our inner voice, we become tuned in to a perfect guide for our body—a guide that will direct us toward certain foods and away from others, and also tell us when we are hungry, when we are full, and when we are just right and in balance.

To Weigh or Not to Weigh

We tend to resist the idea of daily weigh-ins because we are afraid that we will fixate on the number and it will come to rule our lives. And for some of us, this is the absolute truth, and we cannot escape punishing feelings if we are not where we think we are supposed to be on the scale. And if this is the case for you, by all means, avoid daily weigh-ins and instead focus on how you feel and how your clothes fit. Feeling great, after all, is our ultimate goal. But if you are able to do it without judgment or self-condemnation, then regularly weighing yourself may be a helpful exercise. You, and you alone, determine what works best for you.

If you decide to weigh, I suggest getting on the scale every morning as part of your wake-up routine, before you eat anything or get dressed. And if, one morning, you are suddenly five pounds heavier than you were the day before, then you can consider what you ate, and connect the dots, thereby learning something about your body-food connection. Maybe it was sodium that you ate unknowingly, and you are retaining water (Mexican and Chinese foods are both super high in sodium), or maybe it was the second helping or the unusually rich dessert you indulged in. Or if you are down a few pounds, you can consider what you ate in the same manner.

The point is that if we are able to weigh ourselves daily without negative emotional repercussions, we can discover patterns and learn what makes us heavier, and what makes us lighter. It is not the same for everyone. We all process foods differently.

Another advantage of daily weigh-ins is that they help us to maintain our weight once we are where we want to be. If we are up a few pounds, we can bring a little extra awareness and discipline to what we eat throughout the day, knowing that we are on the heavy side. And likewise, if we are down a few pounds, we can indulge a bit where we might not normally. The daily check-in tells us the story when it's still hot off the press.

But I do understand, and understand clearly, that for some of us, it's near impossible to not fixate on the scale in an unhealthy way. In that case, we must learn to be compassionate with ourselves above all else and to honor our individual truth. This is a spiritual journey, after all, and though the scale is not by any means a measure of our worth, I understand that it can, at times, feel that way.

Movement as a Spiritual Practice

Just as our mindful behavior surrounding food becomes a form of spiritual practice because of its intrinsic effect on our health and our feelings of well-being, so too does our behavior surrounding the movement of our bodies. Our emotional well-being can be shifted by varying degrees depending on the state of play in our muscles and our limbs, or the lack thereof. Sedentary bodies suffer for their lack of movement.

Physical equilibrium is equal to spiritual, mental, and emotional equilibrium, and as such, requires that we engage in some kind of daily physical activity beyond the journey back and forth from our cars. And this is true for all of us. Our bodies are meant to move! Done correctly, exercise can change our posture, strength, stamina, and energy. It can alleviate pain. It is an endless resource for self-improvement and evolution. And I could write an entire book on the benefits of stability and core strength and all of the different strategies for reshaping our bodies, but for the purposes of this book, suffice it to say that some kind of everyday movement routine is the essential partner of good health and spiritual fitness.

As a personal trainer, I've witnessed how we tend to overthink the idea of exercise in every way and believe that it has to be a big production involving special clothes, expensive shoes, gyms, aerobic classes, and hours of time out of our week. And if we can afford these things and enjoy them, then all of that is money and time well spent. But if we feel like we have no extra time and minimal motivation, we can still get moving enough to feel good and get our blood circulating.

In the same way that our bodies are intuitive when it comes to food, they have an intuitive movement pattern as well. Some bodies like to jog, some to walk, and some to swim; others do yoga, power-lift, or maybe perform explosive jumps and other maneuvers. We are all a bit different. We need to learn to follow our inclinations and to do what feels good to us so that we keep on doing it. If we are walkers who force ourselves to run, that will likely be unpleasant for us, and we will be less apt to stick with it.

If we are full of excuses and resistance to exercise in general, maybe the best thing we can do for ourselves is to dance in our living rooms, put on some kind of music that we love and move around while it plays in any way that feels good to us. We can dance in hips and hops, long slow flowing moves, gyrations, bumping, grinding, rhythm, swing, country, or disco. It doesn't matter how we move as long as we get moving enough every day to raise our heart rate a bit and get our muscles going for at least a few minutes, and longer if we have the time and the inclination.

I also happen to be a big believer in daily walks. Dogs help us keep on track in this regard, so if we have dogs, all the better. But even without them, we can walk 10 minutes, or 20, or longer as we please. It's good for the body and good for the spirit and satisfies our need for fresh air. In this way, walks are good for the mind as well as the body. They un-stick us when we are stuck and shift our perspective. A good walk opens us to a broader view of things.

Even if we can't walk, or dance, or make any real use of our legs, we can still exercise. We can flop our arms up and down like a bird, conduct like a conductor, extend our fists in front of our chests, rotate our torsos, shake our hands, and turn our heads. We can move whatever moves. "Exercise" can be this simple.

That said, it's no wonder that it still seems daunting to many of us. Perusing the exercise section of any bookstore, or searching the category online, we are confronted with brawny, muscular bodies in impressive poses and postures of all kinds. Ripped, six-pack abs, perfectly toned shoulders, and bulging quadriceps adorn the covers of books and websites. Flipping through pages, we see endless photographs of strong, fit bodies performing all manner of lifts and tilts. And if we are not versed in exercise, these images are likely to intimidate rather than inspire us.

But exercise is for everyone, and it doesn't need to be complicated, beautiful, or driven toward physical perfection and muscular definition. It is simply designed to keep our body in good functioning order. The added benefit is that it makes us feel good: empowered, strong, flexible, and energetic. The fear surrounding exercise is that it will be unpleasant and uncomfortable, and that we will hurt ourselves. We are all familiar with the adage "no pain, no gain," and we fear the pain.

In spite of our fear, exercise can be fun and fulfilling regardless of our fitness level. And we really can keep it as simple as dancing around our living room or taking a daily walk or flopping our arms around like jumping jacks. But if we want to take it one step further, it's useful to understand things at a slightly deeper level.

The Basics of Exercise

If the purpose of exercise is to keep our heart, lungs, muscles, bones, joints, and tendons in good functioning order, then the purpose of daily exercise is to "work out" each of these things. Although we can go to a gym and make this as complicated as we choose to, in its most basic form, a perfectly adequate "routine" doesn't require any large space or special clothing. We can wear our pajamas and slippers and be standing on the kitchen floor. Or we can suit up and head outside—whatever we prefer. The only requirement is that we have an open mind and enough space around us to spread our arms.

We know more about our bodies and our muscles than we think we do. We may not know the exact terminology for things, but we all have a basic, built-in understanding of what's what. Joints allow for the movement of bones. They glide and pivot and hinge and rotate. Ligaments, which are a kind of fibrous tissue, connect bones to each other. Tendons attach muscles to bones, and muscles generate strength and momentum. We can increase the length and power of our muscles, thereby making them more functional, by extending them and contracting, or flexing, them.

This, in turn, creates greater range of motion, greater balance, and greater overall physical health. Our muscles can push, pull, lift, lower, rotate, support, and hold. Using our muscles, we can move forward and backward, side to side, up and down, and in circles.

Our heart is a muscle as well, as are our lungs, but these are "involuntary" as opposed to "voluntary" muscles. They work "by default" at all times, by pumping blood, and converting oxygen, but they *work out* by default, and become stronger, when we use them during exercise.

Our bodies are incredible miracles of design and function. We have more than 200 bones and over 600 muscles. Our hearts beat, our eyes see, our ears hear, and our stomachs digest. But we forget the beauty of our functionality, being consumed as we so often are by the physical-perfection adulation of the culture that we live in. If we do not fit some standardized "norm" of attractiveness, we may feel inadequate. But if we could only muster a bit of genuine appreciation for the wonders of our physical being-ness, it might come easier to believe in our intrinsic value and our endless potential. And to feel better about ourselves on every level.

Exercise can help us to do that. We can learn to enjoy the feeling of our bodies moving and be empowered by the movement. We can become aware of our blood increasing its circulation as we perform simple range-of-motion activities and take pleasure in the increase of warmth and the experience of energy rising within us as we begin our daily routine.

Willingness Exercise: Movement

Performing 5 to 10 minutes of these simple, well-rounded, range-of-motion movements every day can positively affect the quality of your health. You will need a bit of privacy or a willing partner, and an area where you can stand and move your arms up and down and side to side without hitting anything. If you have a medical condition that affects your ability to exercise, be sure to clear these moves with your doctor before performing them. Begin slowly, and make use of modifications as necessary. If you're an avid exerciser, make these moves intense and energetic enough to suit your level of fitness by creating large and expansive ranges of motion.

1. Stand with your feet shoulder-width apart and toes pointing forward, with a slight bend in the knees. Keep your stomach in, chest lifted, and shoulders relaxed.

2. Raise both arms up above your head like you are doing a jumping jack, and then push them down with some intensity. Repeat the move at a fairly quick and steady pace for 15 to 20 fluid repetitions. You can modify the move by performing it from a sitting position, raising only one arm at a time, going slower, doing fewer reps, and not lifting your arms so high overhead. For this, and all successive moves, make sure to make them work for you and your body. Modify them as necessary so that they feel good—these should not be painful—

and feel free to alter them slightly in any way that you like so that you can experience greater comfort.

3. Move your arms straight forward and raise them up in front of you until they are up by your ears—modifying as necessary (see suggestions above)—and then let them drop down and swing behind your back, and then straight back up again, making a forward-backward swinging motion with straight arms. Maintain a fairly quick, steady pace, and repeat for 15 to 20 fluid repetitions. The idea with both of these exercises is to get your heart rate up a bit, so control your pace accordingly. If it is uncomfortable to raise your arms up so high, decrease the range of motion to keep them swinging back and forth below the shoulders.

4. Imagine that you are conducting a large orchestra. With your arms bent slightly at the elbows, bring your hands up together in front of your chest, and then out and wide to the side, squeezing your shoulder blades slightly every time you open wide. Maintain a fairly quick, steady pace for 15 to 20 fluid repetitions and modify as necessary.

5. Stand tall and put your hands on your hips. Lift one knee up toward the ceiling like you're marching in place, and then the other. Continue alternating legs at a fairly

quick and steady pace until you have lifted each leg 15 to 20 times. You can modify the move by holding on to a kitchen counter or the back of a chair for stability, or by lifting your legs lower/higher as it suits you. If you cannot stand on your legs, lift one foot and then the other off of the floor from a sitting position.

6. Keeping the same body position, hands on hips and standing tall, or standing tall while holding on to a chair or counter for support, bend one knee so that your leg lifts up behind you, as if you are going to kick your glutes. Then, repeat the move on the other side and continue to alternate one leg and then the other for a set of 15 to 20 on each leg, keeping a fairly quick and steady pace. Skip this exercise and the two that follow if you are unable to stand up, or else modify them as necessary to manage any pain you may feel in your knees by not lifting as high, etc.

7. Keeping the same body position as the previous exercise, hands on hips and standing tall, or standing tall while holding on to a chair or counter for support, swing one leg forward and backward fluidly like a pendulum, for 10 to 15 swings, and then repeat on the other leg, modifying as necessary for comfort.

8. Continuing in the same body position as the two previous exercises (holding on for support if necessary, but being sure to stand tall and in good posture whether you're holding on or not), raise one leg straight out to the side, as high or low as you are comfortable lifting it, and then switch to the opposite side. Do this at a slow and steady pace, not quite as fast as the others. Repeat 15 to 20 fluid repetitions on each leg.

9. Standing tall, extending your arms loosely out in front of you and clasping your hands together, gently rotate your torso from one side to the other. The motion should be fluid and should not be painful. Start with fairly small rotations and make them bigger as comfort allows. If you are unable to stand, you can perform these rotations from a sitting position.

10. Sitting "perched" on the edge of a chair with your hands on your thighs, lean back slightly until you feel your stomach (abs) tighten. Hold the position for a slow count of 10, or longer if you want to. Keep your chest out and your spine straight, and modify as necessary. The farther you lean back, the more challenging the exercise becomes.

By performing these 10 simple movements, you have touched all of the major muscles in your body, gotten your blood pumping, and done a little bit of weight training as well. Simple, but effective. Exercise can be this easy.

Body Love

If you allowed yourself to relax as you performed the simple exercises above, and modified them as suggested so that you felt no pain and only fluid rhythm, then chances are that you felt warmer when you finished them than when you began, and perhaps even a bit tingly, or energized, as well. Even simple movements can invigorate and uplift us.

It is the vitality of the body that expresses itself through movement, and this vitality is our living energy and life force. Unattended and unappreciated, this energy can become dull and listless. But learning to activate and play with it through movement can help us to feel more alive and more vital, and consequently, more hopeful and full of joy.

Our bodies, like our meals, can become a gateway to enlightenment if we become mindful enough to appreciate them. No matter our exact size or shape, or whatever we might perceive as our physical flaws and imperfections, it's possible to love the solid structure of our flesh and bones. And learning to love our physicality is a good habit and a form of spiritual practice.

We denigrate ourselves and critique our bellies and hips, our balding heads, our shoulders and chins. We are too much of this and not enough of that. We are too tall, too short, too wide, and too scarred. Our hair is too red, too curly, too thin, or too thick; our feet are too long, our arches too high, our eyebrows too bushy. With this kind of thinking, we resist ourselves and miss out on the simple but powerful pleasure of being alive. I am sad for our bodies that we treat them with such loathing and disdain.

But we shouldn't! They house our spirits! And it is our bodies that allow us to experience this incredible world in which we live: the touch of love, the scent of lavender, and the sound of rain on the roof. It is through our bodies that we laugh and cry, listen and sing, watch and learn. We are blessed with respiration, inspiration, digestion, circulation, and sight. We are blessed with the beauty of our skin and the luminescence of our eyes, with red lips and wisps of hair around our face. What gifts these are, and what a gift our body is: a miracle of design and function more complex than any computer and more magnificent than any man-made thing. We have been gifted the experience of living life on this beautiful earth, and we scoff at it. Like whiny children, we are not content.

A celebrated body is a glorious thing, and a maligned body is shrunken and unwell. Our body tells the world how we feel about ourselves. And how we feel about ourselves dictates the way that we experience the world. In the same manner that the food-mood connection travels both ways, with food choices affecting our moods and our moods affecting our food choices, so too, the body-mind-spirit connection travels both ways. If we treat our body with a bit of daily movement and loving thoughts, then we empower our spirits and feel mentally well. And if we empower our spirits by taking responsibility for the care of ourselves, our bodies feel vital and alive. It can come from the outside in or the inside out, but living in a state of wellness requires that we maintain a healthy balance from both sides.

Regarding our bodies, we can err on the side of being too precious and overly protective, afraid that our structure won't hold up, and lacking trust in our physical capabilities. Or we can go to the other extreme and push ourselves physically beyond reason on a daily basis, treating our bodies as if they are indestructible and don't need time for restoration and repair. Either of these positions fails us in the long run, and ultimately, we must learn to listen to the accurate cues from our body. The same voice that tells us when we need to eat, or when we have had enough to eat, also tells us when we need to move or when we need to stop moving. Increasing our appreciation for the wonders of our physical selves and becoming ever more mindful of our moving parts will help us to hear the voice that guides us, and to clearly know what our body wants.

Appreciation Exercise: Your Body, Your Friend

By meditating in the manner suggested, you will feel an increased appreciation for your body. You will need a few minutes of quiet, uninterrupted time and a thoughtful sense of where your body came from; think about who gave it to you and who you have to thank for it. Perhaps you feel that it comes simply from your mother and father, or perhaps, more profoundly, from the Universe, or from God, however, you might understand God. There is no right way to think about this. It is personal to you. But however you think about it, bring that awareness to the forefront of your mind as you perform the exercise below.

If any of your body parts are particularly painful or have caused you difficulty over the years, say thank you as suggested anyway, and send them love, recognizing how you have invested negative energy in their direction.

1. Sit comfortably, with your spine straight, and gently rub your hands together in small circles for about 15 seconds. Then, place your left hand over your heart and your right hand over your left hand, and close your eyes.

2. Bring your attention to your feet and say, "Thank you for my feet." You can say this silently or out loud, whatever feels right to you. And then take a moment to consider the amazing features of your feet: how they move and bend, arch and point, and how you stand on them.

3. Then say, "Thank you for my toes," and consider your toes in the same way. Toes are so much fun! Remember playing "This little piggy went to market," when you were little. Wiggle your toes and appreciate them.

4. Then continue on to your ankles: "Thank you for my ankles." And your calves and shins: "Thank you for my calves and shins." And your knees: "Thank you for my knees."

5. Continue up your body, saying thank you for each part, and considering briefly how it serves you or how you've been hard on it. "Thank you for my hips, thank you for my stomach, thank you for my heart." The idea is to generate love and appreciation and compassion where necessary for the miraculous nature of your physical self.

6. When you have completed the exercise by saying thank you all the way up your body, sit quietly for a moment and tune in to the energy within. Consider whether all of this appreciation has changed the way that you feel, and if so, how?

7. Open your eyes and sit quietly for a minute before you continue on with your day.

Learning to appreciate your body parts in this way can help you raise your level of awareness for the wonderful nature of your functioning parts, and consequently, your level of comfort in your own skin. The result of this awareness is a sense of well-being and profound gratitude that can measurably enrich the quality of your life.

The Importance of Sleep

Our main focus thus far has been in relation to food and exercise, but I want to touch briefly on sleep as well. Like meals and movement, our bodies need daily rest. It's easy to short ourselves in this regard, especially in our fast-paced world with its demanding expectations and so much to do and keep track of. And while I am not convinced that everybody needs eight hours of sleep every night, I am convinced that we all need more than three or four.

Sleep restores and refreshes us. It is our daily healing and recuperation. Without enough of it, we become irritable and overwhelmed by even the simplest of things. So good sleep is an important habit, and it belongs in the spectrum of our well-being. We need it in just the right amount—for us—in order to live the full glory of our enlightened lives.

Review and Daily Action Plan

Good health is largely the result of good habits, and it requires our honest and willing participation on a daily basis. We must commit to the path and be consistent. In order to experience our purest potential, both physically and spiritually, we need to choose our nourishment with care and eat mindfully, savoring every bite.

We need daily movement, regular tuning in to our state of being, the willingness to make changes and adjustments where necessary, and plenty of restorative sleep. Our moods and our equilibrium are directly affected by our diligence in regard to these simple tenets of healthy living, and our skimping on any of them makes for a potentially compromised existence. But why should we settle for mediocrity when, by raising our awareness and claiming responsibility for the condition of our lives, we can enjoy so much more than that? We can experience happiness and satisfaction. We have simply to step up to reality, be sincere, and follow the steps below.

1. Get honest by reducing messy thinking
   into clear and workable statements of truth.

2. Tune in regularly to your inner
   energy and quiet the mind.

3. Identify problematic beliefs and
   behaviors and become willing to change.

4. STOP bad habits and plan in advance.

5. Eat mindfully.

6. Listen for the voice within.

7. Move every day.

8. Appreciate your body!

9. Get enough sleep.

PART TWO

....

LOVE

"A loving heart is the truest wisdom."
—Charles Dickens

This section of the book, "Love," is also divided into two chapters. "Authenticity, Willingness, and Compassion" considers where we stand in relation to the loving relationships in our lives, what our expectations might be of love as a goal and love as a spiritual principle, the importance of personal authenticity, and the fears and limiting beliefs that we may hold, either consciously or unconsciously. The chapter concludes with a willingness exercise that sets us in motion to expand our compassion and appreciation for others, thereby preparing us to experience an ever-higher level of loving energy in our lives.

Chapter four, "Turning Willingness into Love as a Habit," gives us tools for daily practice. With courage and awareness, we consider how to keep ourselves in a state of love readiness, how to grow and maintain the spirit of love on a regular basis, and how to set boundaries where boundaries are necessary, healthy, and for our highest good. Ultimately, by following the suggested path of ongoing willingness as spelled out in this chapter, love becomes a lifestyle, a purpose, a way of being, and a habit; one that will bring us deep satisfaction and sustainable fulfillment in our lives.

CHAPTER THREE

. . . .

Authenticity, Willingness, and Compassion

"We waste time looking for the perfect lover,
instead of creating the perfect love."
—Tom Robbins

Much like our relationship with food, our relationship with love, both as a concept and as a practice, determines our state of well-being in life. As such, it's an important topic, and one not readily discussed except as some kind of pie-in-the-sky romantic fantasy that promises nothing but good feelings and answers all of our prayers and hopes.

But before we get further into the discussion, it's worthwhile and instructive to assess ourselves right up front, to see how we relate to love in general.

Honesty Exercise: Where You Stand with Relationships

Completing the following checklist will help you to take an inventory on how you feel, think, and behave regarding love as it applies in a variety of relationships in your life. The use of the word "love" here refers to a warm and kindly feeling rather than a romantic sentiment. You will need a pen or a pencil and a few minutes of quiet, uninterrupted time.

For each statement below, make a mark in the appropriate column: most of the time, some of the time, or rarely, whichever best applies. Please add any relationships that you feel are important but are not included here.

SELF

Respond to these statements regarding yourself.

	Most of the time	Some of the time	Rarely
• I *feel love* for myself.	____	____	____
• I *think lovingly* about myself.	____	____	____
• I *behave lovingly* toward myself.	____	____	____

PARENTS

Respond to these statements regarding your parents even if they are no longer living.

	Most of the time	Some of the time	Rarely
+ I *feel love* for my mother.	_____	_____	_____
+ I *think lovingly* about my mother.	_____	_____	_____
+ I *behave lovingly* toward my mother.	_____	_____	_____
+ I *feel love* for my father.	_____	_____	_____
+ I *think lovingly* about my father.	_____	_____	_____
+ I *behave lovingly* toward my father.	_____	_____	_____

Spouse or Partner

Leave this blank if you do not currently have a spouse; or, you can complete it in relation to an ex or deceased partner.

	Most of the time	Some of the time	Rarely
+ I *feel love* for my spouse.	____	____	____
+ I *think lovingly* about my spouse.	____	____	____
+ I *behave lovingly* toward my spouse.	____	____	____

Siblings

Consider these statements in regard to all of your siblings in general or contemplate each singly if you prefer. Leave this section blank if you do not have siblings.

	Most of the time	Some of the time	Rarely
+ I *feel love* for my siblings.	____	____	____
+ I *think lovingly* about my siblings.	____	____	____
+ I *behave lovingly* toward my siblings.	____	____	____

FRIENDS

Consider these statements in regard to all of your friends in general or certain ones in particular, whichever you prefer.

	Most of the time	Some of the time	Rarely
• I *feel love* for my friends.	_____	_____	_____
• I *think lovingly* about my friends.	_____	_____	_____
• I *behave lovingly* toward my friends.	_____	_____	_____

WORK

If you do not work, consider these statements in light of your involvement in community service or a church group, book club, or some other regular social interaction.

	Most of the time	Some of the time	Rarely
• I *feel love* for my boss.	_____	_____	_____
• I *think lovingly* about my boss.	_____	_____	_____
• I *behave lovingly* toward my boss.	_____	_____	_____

- I *feel love* for my
  work colleagues.

  _____ _____ _____

- I *think lovingly* about
  my work colleagues.

  _____ _____ _____

- I *behave lovingly* toward
  my work colleagues.

  _____ _____ _____

ACQUAINTANCES

These include familiar cashiers, service personnel, post office workers, etc., that you encounter regularly, but do not really know.

	Most of the time	Some of the time	Rarely
I *feel love* for my acquaintances.	_____	_____	_____
I *think lovingly* about my acquaintances.	_____	_____	_____
I *behave lovingly* toward my acquaintances.	_____	_____	_____

STRANGERS

These are people you encounter in your daily interactions but have never seen before and will likely never see again.

	Most of the time	Some of the time	Rarely
• I *feel love* for strangers.	_____	_____	_____
• I *think lovingly* about strangers.	_____	_____	_____
• I *behave lovingly* toward strangers.	_____	_____	_____

The point of the exercise above is twofold. First, it gives you a measure of your level of comfort, or discomfort, with the idea of love as a common spiritual principle in your life. And secondly, it helps you become familiar with how you may or may not give or withhold love depending on whom you are dealing with. Perhaps you think that your love is to be "reserved" for a few special people in your life and is not for everyone—definitely not for strangers, and possibly not for yourself. There are no right answers here. The purpose is simply to see where you stand.

Nonetheless, it's difficult, if not impossible, to experience love, either intimately, or with others in general, if we do not have a certain amount of basic compassion and appreciation for ourselves. And learning who we are, free from pretense and posturing, is part of the work of love and part of our spiritual journey, and partly what we will address in this chapter. But before we go there, let's consider how it all begins.

In the Beginning

Our first experiences of love come from our parents, and for most of us are probably imperfect at best. We may have been loved with conditions, loved by smothering, loved through discipline, or not loved at all. We may have learned to associate love with abusive cycles or the seeking of approval.

Perhaps our parents were insecure themselves and told us from a young age that we were worthless or gave us that message through actions. Perhaps we were abandoned by our fathers, our mothers, or both of them. Maybe our parents died young and left us to negotiate the world without their influence.

Or maybe we were loved deeply and knew it. Perhaps we were cherished and coddled and given every physical thing that we wanted and needed or could ask for. Or maybe we grew up without anything materially but knew that we were important and valuable because that's what we were told and were shown through affection, kindness, encouragement, and compassion. Everybody's story is different.

But no matter the story, our relationship with our parents is likely to have had its own kinds of pitfalls one way or the other, and I imagine that most of us wished that we had something other than what we got. Our parents were people, after all, just like we are, and they had good days and bad days and all of their own personal anger and fear mixed in with their ability to love.

As children, most of us were probably exposed to some combination of love and heartache—confusing messages of our worth and our worthlessness depending upon our parents' moods and their state of mind on any given day. But at least some of the time, we probably got hugs and kisses from someone: our grandparents, a loving aunt, a nanny, or a family friend, if not our parents themselves. And we probably got some form of punishment as well, and felt every bit of it whether it was physical, emotional, mental, or all of the above.

Because of the convoluted nature of the love that most of us received as children, we learned at a young age to feel fear, shame, and guilt. Something about the way we behaved or the way we were intrinsically seemed to make us lovable or not lovable, and the terms were dictated to us through the behavior of the important adults in our lives, if not their words.

For my part, I got the distinct message as a child that I would be loved as long as I did my best—innocent enough, really, but it set me up for a lifetime of strained effort and over-achievement and feeling like whatever I did was never good enough. I didn't know how to measure my "best." Couldn't I always do better, and then better yet again? I got in the habit of giving everything I had and then some. After a time, this left me worn out and rather used-up feeling.

We all got information about love when we were children from the people of influence who surrounded us. And much of the love that we may have experienced was not really love at all, but rather bargaining and manipulation and maybe even cruelty disguised as goodness.

Meanwhile, in fairy tales, we were exposed to stories like "Cinderella" and "Sleeping Beauty" that told us that we could be "rescued" by romantic love, often in the form of a kiss from a prince and an unlikely chain of events. So many of our childhood epics told us of someone's hard life ending happily ever after because of love. This is reinforced by adult stories with the same plot. As a result, love became for us, at an early age, something distant and far away to be hoped for and blessed with—if we were lucky and beautiful and in the right place at the right time. We began to long for it, and we looked for it in the most unlikely places.

Love is rarely offered up in books and movies as the way for us to be and the thing to do on a daily basis and as a lifetime strategy. Instead, it is just out there, lost and waiting to be discovered, maybe held captive by a spell; it is not within us at all but encapsulated in some kind of "other" person—some hero or victor or fairy-tale prince.

So it's no wonder that when we became teenagers and started to feel drawn to others in a physical way, that we were certain it must be the lure of love. Our time had come at last to be the prince or the princess. We entered into a kind of love-hunt and looked for it everywhere. And we put up with endless nonsense and dysfunction believing in the magic of our childhood stories. I got the idea somehow that the more troubled an individual was, the more likely they embodied the love that I hoped for, and I was always on the lookout for toads I could kiss.

Expectations Versus Reality

We expect another person to fulfill us and to bring us love and to make us feel the loving feeling. We expect another person to be our happily ever after, to right our wrongs and make okay all of our childhood horror—to end once and for all the evil rule of our wicked stepmother. But another person can't do that. No matter how much we want them to and believe in them, another person can't fix what ails us. Only we can do that. Doing that is our job and our journey.

And doing that—fixing ourselves—is part of love. It's an important part, maybe the most important part. It comes before everything else. As mentioned earlier, we cannot be in a healthy, loving relationship with anyone else until we know how to behave in a healthy and loving manner toward ourselves.

On some level, this is a familiar concept. We have all encountered one version of it or another, but it's still difficult to understand. What does it mean to love ourselves? Isn't it selfish to do so? Isn't it wrong? Aren't we supposed to be all about everyone else and making sure that the people we care about are happy and taken care of and well fed? Isn't that our primary duty in a love relationship?

Certainly that's what many of us have been told, often enough that we now believe it. Consequently, we don't understand when the people we fuss over don't seem to appreciate our efforts—our children, spouses, parents, and friends. We are doing everything right. We are giving so much. Why don't they fall at our feet in adoration and gratitude? And how is it that they can actually appear hostile and annoyed with us at times in the face of our incomparable generosity?

We are actually smothering them like this, and it becomes a vicious cycle. They lash out in frustration, which makes us do more, and makes them feel more smothered. They say they can't breathe, and we don't understand. They resent our unending attention and we resent their lack of appreciation. I have been at both ends of this game, and neither one is particularly satisfying or fun.

One of the most difficult concepts to understand and integrate is that love is letting go. We have no doubt heard this before, but how are we supposed to do it? All of our instincts tell us to hold on to the ones we love no matter what, to be there for them constantly, to enmesh our lives with theirs, and to be each other's everything.

But this kind of entwined existence, especially in intimate relationships, is not usually love so much as it is codependence, and it is rooted in fear. It tells us that we cannot survive without the other, that we need the relationship, that our hearts would break and we would be lost and devastated if anything happened to our partner or to our love. Yet, things happen to loves like this all the time. One or the other partner gets to a place where they just can't stand it anymore. It feels like a form of entrapment, and the one who is left can hardly function alone and is miserable, bereft, and victimized until he or she realizes that the other person is not a requirement for happiness.

We have to learn how to be okay on our own if we ever want to feel the deep completion and pure connection of true love that allows for space and movement. But more often than not, a person such as the one described above just moves on to another relationship with all of the same enmeshing qualities and continues in this cycle ad infinitum, trying to get it right each successive time by giving more and enmeshing more; however, "more" doesn't usually work out any differently than it did the first go-round.

Still, others do fine under the model described above. They become completely dependent upon each other and it somehow works for them. They go everywhere together, do everything together, finish each other's sentences, and carry on this way for years. They become a kind of force field of established routines and structures and are a complete universe in and of themselves. It's them against the world, and that's the way they like it.

But I would argue that such a situation is maybe more about attachment and habit than it is about love, and might not really be for the highest good of the individuals involved or the community at large. It functions, but may not be entirely healthy. It is diminishing rather than enlarging, and limited by its own design.

The bottom line is that we all have certain ideas and expectations about what role love is supposed to play in our lives. And these expectations are important because they may be the very thing that ends up limiting us, and blocking us from the reality of love in the end.

Awareness Exercise:
Expectations and What You Believe

This exercise is designed to help you see how far apart your expectations of love are from your actual experience. You will need a pen or a pencil and a few minutes of quiet, uninterrupted time. Complete the two statements by circling all that apply.

1. *Love is supposed to (be)…*

easy	magical	perfect
special	fulfilling	natural
freeing	unconditional	accepting
beautiful	difficult	scary
confusing	suffocating	conditional
unfair	judgmental	ordinary
given to me	my responsibility	make me happy

| answer my prayers | my life purpose | free me from pain |
| for everyone | reserved for special people | for only the lucky |

2. *Love is actually…*

easy	magical	perfect
special	fulfilling	natural
freeing	unconditional	accepting
beautiful	difficult	scary
confusing	suffocating	conditional
unfair	judgmental	ordinary
given to me	my responsibility	make me happy
answer my prayers	my life purpose	free me from pain
for everyone	reserved for special people	for only the lucky

Consider how the two completed lists are different and how they are the same. The more dramatic the dichotomy, the more likely you are to feel a certain dissatisfaction with love in your life. A sense of well-being comes when you can honestly respond to this exercise and discover that for the most part, both lists match.

Potential and Discernment

So how do we go about defining love? Does it have certain characteristics that we can systematically pinpoint? Can dysfunctional love still be love? Is the love we feel for some people different from the love that we feel for others? Or does all love ultimately come from the same source? And if so, what is that source? There are lots of questions but no agreed-upon answers.

In my experience, love is living energy that comes into the world through us. And when it comes through, it is pure. But depending upon what it encounters, it can be reflected back to us with equivalent purity or become warped and twisted and tangled up with fear. So who we give our love to matters in terms of the love we feel coming back to us in return. When we're young and looking for our love savior, we are willing to offer it up to anyone who seems at all interested in what we have to give, which makes us potential victims of dangerous others. We may attract people to us who do not have our best interests in mind. For this reason, age is a blessing because we learn over time who has the ability to love us, and not merely the potential.

Potential is an interesting and intriguing concept. Though we all, certainly, have the innate potential to be loving and to experience all of the blessings and benefits of great love, the truth is that not all of us reach this potential. Those individuals who are on the self-actualizing path often assume that everyone else is traveling the same road toward fulfillment; yet, if we take the time to consider it honestly, we know that this is not necessarily the case.

Some die before reaching their potential and some never even bother trying to reach it. This is an unfortunate, but true, fact. And yet, for the hopeful among us, it's easy—too easy almost—to fall in love with who someone *could be* instead of who they actually are. Many of us do this, especially when we are young. We see possibility in our prospective lovers and know how incredible they would be if they just made this simple change—or that one. We make the fairy-tale error of believing that our love can, and will, be the thing to bring them around.

We have to be realistic about who we're dealing with. We project ourselves onto others and assume that they will react as we would react, and feel as we feel. And some sympathetic others may do just that, but most do not. In Ayn Rand's book *Atlas Shrugged*, one of her main characters, Dagny Taggart, has exactly this problem as described in the introduction to the thirty-fifth anniversary edition: "Her error is over-optimism. She thinks...she can make people do what she wants or needs, what is right, by the sheer force of her own talent; not by forcing them, of course, not by enslaving them and giving orders—but by the sheer over-abundance of her own energy; she will show them how, she can teach them and persuade them, she is so able that they'll catch it from her."

Much as we have to learn how to love and how to be loving, we have to learn how to discern and how to be discerning: how to see clearly. The art of clear sight is the result of experience. In youth for sure, and sometimes well into our lives, most of us are completely blind to the truth of who is before us. We see what we want to see, and fall in love with our projected fantasies. And then we are crushed when our fantasies crumble before us. No one is more surprised than we are when our dreams of ardor crash to the ground.

Compassion and Appreciation

The evolved journey is to see what is, to see who is actually there, and to love and appreciate that. We need to understand that we can only experience an exchange of love when love is what's before us. Otherwise what we might actually be engaging in under the guise of love are mind-games and codependency at best, and sexual addiction and abuse at worst. When we believe these things are love, we end up feeling fiercely let down.

Real love is about real appreciation, which is full of patience, forgiveness, and compassion. Such a love requires that we understand the actual value of a person and have a desire to do no harm to that person but to celebrate them and honor them as they are, with all of their limitations. And in an ideal situation, love completes itself by having this same kind of appreciation returned in kind.

Having the energy of real love moving through us results in a good feeling, a "loving" feeling, and when we are "in love" we are almost euphoric from just how good we feel. But sadly, for most of us, it doesn't seem to last. It seems to have a kind of on-again off-again pattern in which we feel "in love" much of the time, as if nothing can go wrong and life is beautiful and blissful, and then without warning we feel unsure, and almost dark, as if everything could go wrong.

I would argue that we unconsciously flip-flop from love to fear and back again over and over for the bulk of our lives. And I would further argue that all of it begins in us—not in the other person and not in the world at large. We don't get our loving feeling from another person; we get it from the compassion and the appreciation for life and for others that starts inside of us.

But love has layers and heights that go above and beyond any earthly description, or even any attempt at description. Love is cosmic and divine, something bigger than we are or than we can completely comprehend. I believe love is the most powerful force on earth and the answer to any and all of our questions. And that when we are "in love," whether because of a person or a beautiful vista or a sense of well-being, then everything is beautiful and we begin at those moments to "get it" in the big sense of the word "it."

"It" in this sense is all-inclusive. It is purpose and plan and perfection. So in this bigger sense of the word, I believe love is transcendent. But whatever it is exactly, or however we might characterize it, hopefully we can all agree that love is something we need and something we want, even if we don't, or won't, admit it. And hopefully, we can also agree that love has something to do with compassion and something to do with appreciation: an understanding and valuing of others and an understanding and valuing of ourselves.

Authenticity

So in order for us to experience love in the biggest and best way possible, where and how do we begin? The easy answer is from wherever we are and with absolute honesty. And we have already started that process in the exercises we have completed. What comes next is to consider what we find lovable in others. What inspires in us the compassionate appreciation that we have described above?

More than material things and impressive statistics, I believe we feel natural, outpouring love for others when we experience their authenticity. We can appreciate their expertise and the curve of their lips and bodily stature, but in my experience, our love is for their lack of pretense; for their struggling and beautiful spirit as it rises above the challenges of daily life; and for the raw presence of their absolute truth. This is what inspires compassion and appreciation in us.

And sometimes this truth is their vulnerability, and sometimes it is the perfect and sublime expression of their divine gift. We witness their authenticity, but we also participate in it. Authenticity in others inspires authenticity in us. It gives us permission to be who we are without pretense, and a kind of union occurs. Duality disappears and we no longer feel separate from each other. We feel connection and oneness.

Webster's defines authenticity as "trustworthy and genuine; corresponding to truth: being actually and precisely what is claimed." By its very definition, it is rooted in honesty. So being authentic is being honest with others and with ourselves as well as being honest about our victories, failures, fears, motivations, and limitations. Authenticity accepts the good and the bad. It celebrates wholeness and does not apologize for itself. It is pure expression of the energies of life. And the result of authenticity is love. It sees beyond the surface to the truth within.

If love is hidden, then it's hidden right in front of our eyes. It is inside people and inside of us. It is in the way we express ourselves and show the world who we are underneath. And yet, we spend time and effort developing masks, fortresses, and walls so that no one can see us—and so no one does. And then we wonder why we don't feel love. We block others from seeing it in us, and consequently, we become incapable of seeing it in ourselves.

If we want to experience love in our lives, we must become willing to be at least somewhat see-through. We must let down our barriers and expose our authentic selves to the world and be willing to be vulnerable and imperfect—exactly who we are without any kind of facade. This kind of willingness in an ongoing way requires great courage, but before the courage, we need simply the willingness. And we can build that up as a kind of spiritual habit.

Willingness Exercise: Embracing Your Authentic Self

By regularly repeating the affirmation below—in the morning when you wake up, in the evening before sleep, and whenever you think of it throughout the day—you will increase your ability to be authentic and true to yourself, which helps you more effectively experience love in your life. You will need a pen or pencil, your journal, and a few quiet, uninterrupted moments.

Read the passage below out loud to yourself several times. Go slowly and really feel each statement as you read through. Then pick the sentence, or statement, that resonates most strongly with you and write it in your journal in large letters. This is your affirmation. Commit it to memory, and repeat it as suggested above.

+ *I am willing to be exactly who I am. I am willing to accept myself with all of my gifts and imperfections. I am willing to share myself with the world. I am willing to stop pretending that I am something other than I am. I am willing to drop all pretense. I am willing to be vulnerable. I am willing to admit that I am good at some things, and not so good at others. I am willing to be emotional, and to show my emotions. I am willing to feel good about myself. I am willing to be okay with the fact that I can't do everything and be everything to everyone all of the time. I am willing to communicate honestly about what's going on inside of me. And I am willing to believe that I am lovable no matter what.*

With this kind of willingness, we can change our lives for the better. Willingness is powerful medicine. It awakens spiritual energy within us that begins the expansion of love in our lives.

Identifying Blocks

One practical result of our willingness is a raised awareness regarding how we may have become habituated to blocking love in our lives. Love can be blocked in many ways and on many levels. It is blocked by resentment, anger, fear, insecurity, and greed; by guilt and shame, economics, politics, prejudice, and habit.

And perhaps, more than anything else, we are blocked by our own limiting beliefs and expectations, some of which we identified in the "What You Believe" exercise earlier in this chapter. Perhaps we expect that we will never find love, that we don't deserve love, or that we have to earn love by good behavior or by looking or being a certain way. Or maybe we tell ourselves that we don't believe in love at all, that it's something for the movies but not for real life, and definitely not for us. Knowing what we believe and expect erroneously about love makes it easier to recognize when it bubbles up, and we can learn to dispel it with compassion, to shift our perspective, and to change our point of view.

Our self-consciousness is another barrier to love. If we feel awkward, unworthy, unattractive, or unwell; if we are blind with self-pity or doubt ourselves at every turn, it's nearly impossible to be open to loving energy, even if it's right in front of us. This tendency toward negative self-absorption can become a habit, and a powerful one. But we can shift it slowly over time. By raising our awareness and engaging our willingness, we can become diligent lookouts for this negative trend. We can learn to watch for it sneaking up quietly, like a tiger in the brush.

Blocks to love will inevitably rise and fall within us like the tides for as long as we live, but we can get better and better at identifying when we are blocked and why.

The Drawbridge of Love

Love is somewhat like a drawbridge. We raise it and lower it as we choose. And when we are blocked, our drawbridge is stuck in the drawn-up position, so nothing can come to us. From our guarded position, fortressed and secure, we may be able to fire off cannons at others but we cannot send out love—not until we are willing to lower our drawbridge. And some people never do.

Lowering the drawbridge takes the courage and willingness to be vulnerable that we have previously discussed. It requires that we trust ourselves and that we trust others, at least a little bit. But what glory and delight if we meet others whose drawbridges are also down. We can have a love exchange! We can share a smile or a laugh or a story or lots of stories. We can take a walk and appreciate the natural and beautiful world in which we live. We can eat a meal together with pleasure. We can share our wounds and our hopes. And the whole time, loving energy is passing back and forth between us. And it feels good and uplifts our spirits and gives us the sense that we belong and that we matter.

And hopefully we can learn to go along in life mostly open, mostly authentic, and mostly willing to let our love go out, and to freely take it in. But without a doubt, we will encounter many who are shut tight, like doors. And every time we face them, we have a choice. We can give them love anyway, and hope a little of it slips around the edges, or we can defensively shut our own doors and pull up our own bridges. That's the instinctual response. When facing anger, or anything unpleasant in others, we have a tendency to retreat.

But we don't have to. We can understand that angry and upset people are actually crying out for love, and we can choose to be kind to them. We can be authentically loving toward others even if they are incapable of loving us back, whether permanently or temporarily. We can accept that they are where they are, and that it's not personal to us. We can have compassion knowing that we go there ourselves every now and again, and that sometimes we get stuck there too. But love can still reach us even if we are hostile toward its advances. It can and does creep through the cracks and shine its light across the darkness.

Awareness Exercise: Opening to Love

By curling and tightening your body and your muscles as described below, you will experience metaphorically what happens to your energy when you are blocked to love. By releasing tension, you will understand what happens when you make the decision to open up. You will need a few quiet, uninterrupted moments and a chair.

1. Sit comfortably, but in good posture, and
   close your eyes. Take a few long, slow breaths.

2. Cross your legs and your arms, make fists of
   your hands, tuck your chin, round your back,
   and clench your jaw, squeezing all of your muscles,
   and pulling yourself into a tight ball. Hold this
   position long enough to feel how uncomfortable
   it is—30 seconds, a minute?

3. Visualize yourself as love personified, hiding in an
   uncomfortably small space, afraid of being discovered.

4. Slowly, and consciously, release your muscles.
   Imagine love becoming curious and willing,
   poking a head around the corner, coming out
   of hiding and into the light. Straighten your spine,
   open your arms, uncross your legs, sit upright
   again, and relax. Take a few long, slow breaths.

The key to recognizing when we are blocked to love in our lives is to become aware of physical or energetic "tightening" and rigidity. And the opening process, just like in this exercise, is simply a conscious decision to relax and let go.

Accepting Ourselves as We Are

The journey to experiencing love in our lives is a journey of remembering our own loveliness, and then being able to recognize that same loveliness in others—something easily forgotten and overlooked as we strive for success and struggle to make ends meet and to get along. But we can do better than that, and we need to if we want to live our best lives. Our birthright is love and our birthright is beauty and grace. We deserve these things. But they will not come to us if we are not willing to claim our part in the exchange.

It starts when we become willing to be authentically ourselves. When we stop pretending that we are something other than what we are and stop maintaining elaborate facades, energy is released within us that would otherwise be strained and rigid. This release of tension is the loosening of love, and the opening of a symbolically clenched fist. Such release and relaxation represents our acceptance of ourselves with all of our imperfections. We have nothing to apologize for, or to shrink from.

Living in the open air of acceptance and authenticity and having the ongoing willingness to show our true selves to the world keeps loving energy flowing from us, and consequently, to us. But life happens, and fear rises, and we will draw up into ourselves. It's inevitable that this will happen. We will raise our drawbridge. We will pull back from life like a turtle retreating into his shell. Of course, there are times and places where self-protection is advisable and necessary, but retreat may not always be our best strategy, as it isolates us, and tends to hold us in fear. We will consider methods for appropriate boundary-setting further in the next chapter.

For now, suffice it to say that maintaining an ongoing willingness to be our authentic selves no matter what is the continual work of love preparedness. And catching ourselves when we have retreated in error or for too long, and willingly coming forth into the world authentically again and again, is the continuing journey.

Once our willingness to accept our own vulnerability has been somewhat mastered, then we can willingly accept and appreciate the vulnerability of others. The one follows naturally from the other. We learn compassionate appreciation for ourselves first and then we have compassionate appreciation for others. Having and growing this outpouring compassion is a key tenet of the experience of love in our lives. We have to give it away to keep it.

Appreciation Exercise: Compassion for Others

By learning to look for signs of vulnerability in people's faces, as this exercise suggests, you will raise your ability to feel and experience compassion. You will need four pictures of regular people of varying ages and races who are not famous or known to you in any way. Google Images is a good source for locating such pictures. You can search "average people," and find a wide selection to choose from.

1. Sit quietly, in good posture, and close your eyes. Take a few long, slow breaths and let go of any tension you may feel. If your shoulders are tight, say, "My shoulders are relaxing." Say this over and over until you can feel

them letting go. And then repeat this in regard to any area where you feel tension. Say, "My neck is relaxing; my lower back is relaxing; my hands are relaxing," and continue to say these things until you feel your muscles loosening and a quiet feeling of peace overtake you. Throughout this process of releasing and relaxing your muscles, imagine yourself opening to the energy of love.

2. Look at the first picture with the idea of compassion in your mind rather than judgment. Observe the person's facial features and take note of any signs of strain or sadness around the eyes or elsewhere. Look for wrinkles, imperfections, scars—signs of life having been lived. Observe your reaction to the picture, your possible inclination to judge, to criticize, or to second-guess. Imagine what it might be like to be this person, how it might feel to be inside his body, her face. Imagine him/her trying really hard to be liked, longing for love, and feeling insecure and afraid. Feel compassion for the ways this individual may have suffered in his or her life. And then, in parting, send the person love and blessings, in whatever manner feels right to you.

3. Repeat the exercise with each of the three remaining pictures.

Understanding and appreciating that as human beings, we all suffer with spiritual, mental, emotional, and physical aches and pains, insecurities, unfulfilled hopes and dreams, and our share of grief and loss, it becomes easier to have compassion for each other. Not one of us is immune to these things, no matter how shiny and bright our exteriors may appear. And recognizing the vulnerability in all of us makes for a kinder and gentler path through life. This is the way of shared experience and connection. And this is the way of love.

CHAPTER FOUR

· ·

Turning Willingness into Love as a Habit

> "Love doesn't sit there like a stone, it has to be
> made like bread; remade all the time, made new."
> —Ursula K. Le Guin

Through exercises and discussion in the last chapter, we have grown our awareness and our willingness to be authentic and vulnerable and found ways to identify the presence of limiting beliefs and things that block us to love. In this chapter, we step up. We take action and establish new habits in order to actualize love in our lives on a daily basis and in an ongoing way. This takes courage.

Willingness Exercise:
Visualization for Becoming Courageous

By visualizing yourself being connected solidly to the earth and sky, you feel powerful and brave, and understand that you are stronger than you realize. You will need a few moments of quiet, uninterrupted time.

1. Sit quietly with good posture: your feet flat on the floor and your hands resting on your thighs, palms down. Close your eyes and take a few long, slow breaths.

2. Visualize yourself standing on top of a mountain with a commanding view. You have a wide stance and a spear in your right hand that is resting on the ground beside you and pointing skyward. You are standing tall, your shoulders are broad, and your chest and head are held high. Wind is blowing all around you, but you are standing fast.

3. Visualize cables, streams of light, or roots growing out of your feet and extending all the way to the center of the earth, grounding you solidly where you stand. Visualize the same cables or streams of light extending upwards from the top of your head and rising into the sky, connecting you to the air, to spirit, and to light.

No matter how hard the wind may blow around you, you are connected and supported. You have the earth solidly beneath you and the sky above. You are centered and stable and strong. And no matter what direction you may choose to move, you maintain these connections. You are bigger than you might seem at first glance. You are earth and light, human and spirit, worldly and divine: irrepressible, immovable, and sure.

Taking Responsibility

Being authentic does not mean that we are weak, it means that we are real. We can be vulnerable, but we needn't be victims. It is our job to take responsibility for the condition of our inner selves at any and all times. The idea is to be strong and tender at the same time, and in appropriate ways. We need some toughness in order to be assertive and to set boundaries, but we have to maintain a loving heart. We must learn to be kind and compassionate, yet firm. Real gentility is strength subdued and softness by choice. It is not voluntary weakness.

This idea is aptly demonstrated in the Aesop's fable about the sun and the wind who compete with each other to see who can get a man to remove his coat. The wind pummels him with all of its brute force, but this only makes the man pull his coat in closer and tighter. The sun, on the other hand, is gentle, warm, and persuasive; unquestionably powerful but encouragingly patient, and the sun ultimately convinces the man to take off his coat.

In this way, we can clear ourselves of the things that block us to love. We cannot attack ourselves with forceful winds of anger or intensity, but must be like the sun—intentionally gentle, compassionate, patient, smiling, and warm. We must be courageous in our honesty and aware of our tendency to cave in and shut tight.

The practical side of clearing blocks is to catch ourselves in the act of harsh and critical thoughts and negative behaviors, and be willing to change. When we call ourselves idiots, we can hear ourselves do it and stop. We can change the word and change the energy. We can "flip the script." We are clearly not idiots. Maybe we were trying to do too much at once and made a mistake in our haste. We can tell ourselves to take a deep breath and slow down. Rather than lashing ourselves with negative judgment, we can reassure ourselves that it's okay and we have more time than we think. This is the loving way.

Forgiveness

Generally speaking, when we are feeling hateful, either with ourselves or others, we have become stuck in fear. I like to think of love and fear as the two main baskets of emotions that we experience. In the love basket is gratitude, happiness, tolerance, forgiveness, joy, excitement, and other positive, good-feeling emotions. And in the fear basket is suspicion, anger, impatience, resentment, shame, and greed, to name just a few.

When we are full of negativity and living from the fear side of the equation, there is a process by which we can make the shift back to love. For the purposes of our discussion, we have been calling this process "clearing our blocks." We touched on it briefly in the previous section, but we need to understand it in more depth and detail if we want to make it a positive habit and an effective tool in our lives.

There are three steps to the process: identification, consideration, and resolution. We begin by acknowledging, or identifying, that we feel out-of-sorts. It's possible that we can pinpoint an exact event or moment that "made us mad," or "stressed us out," or something specific that we are afraid of, or feel guilty about; but it's equally possible that we have no idea what is causing our irritation. The purpose of the first part of the block-clearing process is simply to identify that we feel blocked.

The second step is to consider the cause. If we know what it is immediately, all the better, but if we are unsure, this is the time to do a bit of self-reflective trolling for information. We think when we were last feeling good and remember the events that followed. Sometimes it becomes clear upon review what has upset us, and sometimes it's not so obvious. Often, our own less-than-admirable behavior has triggered us and we are feeling shameful and self-conscious, or we may have a kind of free-floating fear of some upcoming event or simply be overwhelmed with exhaustion. Without holding ourselves to perfectionist standards, in this step we do the best we can to understand why we are feeling "off."

The third step is resolution in the form of compassion, forgiveness, and making amends. We are human, and therefore, fallible. And so is everyone we encounter on a daily basis. We cannot hold ourselves or anyone else to standards and expectations that are impossible to meet—not if we want to feel loving and happy. We must forgive ourselves for being less than perfect, for having negative emotions, for speaking when we might have done better to remain quiet, for losing our temper, and for being occasionally unkind. And we have to forgive others for the same things.

We have a tendency to hold a resentment if someone snaps at us, doesn't properly acknowledge or appreciate us, or whatever it may be that causes us to be upset on any given day. And yet, if we're honest, we can fairly easily discover some moment in our own history when we did the same thing to someone else. To forgive is to give up our claim to righteousness. It's to live and let live; to allow for the fallibility in ourselves and others on a regular basis and as a daily practice.

Refusing to forgive sets us up in permanent negativity and blocks us to the experience of love. It sets us apart and makes us feel superior to others, or inferior to them, depending, even though neither viewpoint is true. There is freedom in understanding that it's okay for us to make mistakes of all kinds, and that it is normal and appropriate that we do so, and that others do so as well. It's part of the human condition. Living in the open air of love and forgiveness is good living, and it's our best option for fulfillment and satisfaction in life.

But our forgiveness doesn't end up meaning much if we continue to make the same mistakes over and over. We have to own our part in creating negative drama and take responsibility for our actions. So there is a finishing step of resolution, and that is to say we're sorry to someone we may have wronged, and then do better going forward. We have to make a commitment to improve our behavior. We have to learn from our errors and then demonstrate our learning by acting differently the next time around.

Willingness Exercise: Catching Yourself

By following the block-clearing process described above, and spelled out below, you will be able to restore yourself to feelings of love and well-being whenever you feel troubled. This exercise is designed as a daily practice and an ongoing life skill. You will need the willingness to be self-reflective and use your best observational skills.

1. Identify when you feel rigidity, tension, strong displeasure, or any kind of disturbance, either mentally, emotionally, or physically.

2. Consider the cause, whatever it may be. Perhaps you have been triggered negatively by a conversation, an interaction, or something you have done; maybe you saw something in a magazine or online or began obsessing about the future or regretting the past. As we know from our food journaling, sometimes our discomfort is the result of being hungry. But we are more interested here with feelings that shut you down rather than blood sugar–related mood swings.

Keep in mind that *someone* cannot be the cause of your angst, though what someone said, or did, may trigger feelings in you that create emotional stiffening, or tightening. It is the triggered feelings we are interested in here—not the other person's behavior.

3. Resolve your upset with compassion and forgiveness, for yourself, and anyone else who has played a part. Acknowledge where errors in judgment, perception, and action have been made, and then say out loud, or silently to yourself, that you forgive the wrongdoing. These can be small or large errors. Forgiveness works the same on both.

Scenarios

+ I forgive myself for gossiping in the break room today after lunch.

+ I forgive my boss for not acknowledging my birthday.

+ I forgive myself for overstepping my bounds and trying to control my friend.

+ I forgive my spouse for being short with me and hurting my feelings.

+ I forgive myself for being rude to the cashier.

+ I forgive myself for having unrealistic expectations of my parents.

- I forgive my brother for not inviting me to come along.

4. Apologize to anyone you may have wronged and learn from the experience. Resolve to do better in the future by acting differently and reacting differently.

5. Make this process a habit.

Using this exercise to learn to clear what blocks you and regularly forgiving yourself and others for errors of all kinds, is a practical as well as a spiritual habit. It increases the loving energies of appreciation and compassion and allows for resentment-free living.

Intimate Relationships

To this point, our discussion has been about love in a generalized sense: characteristics of love, love for ourselves and for others, how it can be blocked within us, and how it needs to be regularly cleared. Let us turn now to the more specific topic of successful and healthy interpersonal love relationships. These are particularly sought after and particularly high in their rate of failure. Why should that be?

For starters, it's not possible to have a healthy and functional loving relationship when one or both partners are chronically blocked to love, or when one or both partners have their drawbridges locked fast in the up position and are all about defensiveness and garrisons. Healthy intimacy requires loving energy to flow back and forth.

Plenty of dysfunctional intimate relationships exist, and most of us have probably been in at least one of these in our lifetime. For my part, I have been in many. But I didn't get to experience real love, no matter how loving I felt, until I encountered another individual who was committed to love as a principle and love as a concept in his own life.

Secondly, the journey to a healthy, loving intimate relationship begins with healthy relating to ourselves. We must learn the art of care and kindness before we can give it away. We must learn compassion and self-honesty and appropriate boundaries and communication. These things, in whole or in part, may come naturally to some people, but in my experience, they do not come naturally to most. So we have to learn about them and learn how to integrate them into our lives.

But even if we have attained our full capacity of vibrant loving energy, we cannot head out into the world and have a loving exchange with anyone we choose. Whether we are male or female, if we choose our potential partner because of their looks, their jobs, their family background, or their education, we will likely not find what we are hoping for. Our radar must be tuned to those who have loving energy, who are willing to listen and talk and share from the heart, who show compassion, who take good care of themselves, and who have a gentleness about them even if they are physically strong.

We are steered astray by our upbringings. We look on the surface and determine value with our eyes and our minds instead of our hearts. We think physical strength in a man promises us protection and that beauty in a woman promises us desire, but this is not necessarily so. What attracts us over and across time is *inner* beauty and the energy of love.

So that is what we're looking for, and that is what we want to open ourselves up to. That is where we will find pleasure and laughter and long-term satisfaction—not in fancy cars and big houses and expensive clothes, but in kindness and freedom and acceptance of who we are. Loving people have the ability to love us because they love themselves. Unloving people do not. It's really that simple.

The "work" of love, or love in action, is all about the ongoing desire to evolve, to improve, to follow our True North and our true purpose, both as individuals and together as a couple. Love is letting go in the sense that it cannot hold the beloved back. It must encourage her forth and support him on his path. Wherever we may be called or led in terms of our life purpose, our partner cannot ceaselessly resist us, or we will depart. We have to believe in and support each other.

A relationship that is rooted in healthy and sincere love is not all about one partner making it big or living his dream, but about both partners supporting each other. It recognizes the unique and intrinsic value of the individuals, what each has to offer the world, and what each has to express. And it also recognizes the value of the partnership itself as an entity. What characteristics does the union feature? Is it inspiring to others? Is it supportive of any children? Is it growing? Is it grounded in good communication?

So often, we settle far short of this. We get married and become uninteresting. We stop talking to each other and cease to be excited about possibilities that abound. We plop in front of the same television shows week after week and live vicariously though our favorite television personalities.

We need to invest time, energy, and enthusiasm in our intimate relationships and not allow them to wither or bog down. We do this by taking responsibility for keeping ourselves inspired and refreshed by life and encouraging our partners to do the same. Our purpose is to expand and evolve, not to settle. But we have a role in this. We may need to change some of the familiar ways we go about things in order to properly habituate ourselves to love as a daily experience. We need to raise it up inside ourselves and grow it from within. Then we can inspire it in others and enjoy our intimate relationships, and all of our relationships, free from toxic negativity.

Willingness Exercise: Daily Practice for Growing Love

By focusing on what you love and what's positive and beautiful in yourself and in others, you can change your life for the better, become a more loving individual, and almost instantaneously shift your mood. All you need is the willingness to begin.

1. Identify things that you feel loving toward and express your feelings either out loud or silently to yourself. Start anywhere. Look around and find things that you love.

2. Master this exercise and make it a regular habit.

Example #1

I love the color yellow. I love pine trees. I love silence and just the right amount of wind. I love mountains. I love feeling cozy. I love heat on a cold day and ice-cold water when it's hot. I love to watch bunches of birds in flight patterns overhead and the feeling of being done with work at the end of a long day. I love candlelight, sunlight, and firelight. I love dawn and dusk and the full moon. I love to sleep and to wake up.

It's this simple—not complicated at all—but quite profound in its effect. This practice stirs up love and gets it moving. And once it's moving, it can flow out and around and make you feel good, and make others feel good too!

Another daily practice to grow love is to finish "I am" statements in a loving manner. Language is a strong force for programming change within, and the two words "I am" are creative and powerful beyond measure.

There is a profound difference between the energy of saying "I am ugly and fat and no one will ever love me," and "I am beautiful." Likewise, there is a difference between the very common, "I am bored," and "I am vital and alive." If you live in the breezes of negative self-expression you will feel negative, and vice versa.

3. Complete "I am" statements in a positive and loving way, and do this as a regular habit. You can speak out loud or silently to yourself, in front of a mirror or not, as you please.

Example #2

I am full of goodness. I am kind. I am healthy. I am considerate. I am an excellent friend. I am strong and organized and capable. I am happy. I am blessed. I am in love with my husband. I am renewed every day.

Again, it's not complicated. Anytime and anywhere, we can make these statements to ourselves, and if we're really feeling it, we can share them with others and lift their spirits as well. "You are beautiful. You are smart. You are graceful. You are wise." We can include each other. We can expand our enthusiasm and good feelings outward. Doing this is fun, and we can't lose. It's a win-win proposition.

Simple but Not Easy: The Importance of Boundaries

If we have the courage to be authentically ourselves, keep an eye out for what blocks us, develop positive self-talk and positive behavior habits, and refuse to overcomplicate things in our minds, we can grow love in our lives. We can look for loveliness everywhere, and if we're looking for it, we will find it. It seems almost impossibly simple, but over time, with our consistent attention, we will begin to feel more love, both for ourselves and for the people we encounter.

And as we become more loving, we attract more love. We have an open drawbridge and an open door. And this is a beautiful thing. But if love is unfamiliar territory for us, we must proceed with caution. Newly grown love within us is like a sprouting plant. It needs care and protection. We must learn to watch out for those who would take advantage of our happiness and effervescence.

I used to give my love recklessly. I assumed that everyone wanted what was best for me because I wanted what was best for them, and it all felt like a happy love party with nothing but good feelings and warm fuzzies. I was like a dog wagging my tail and wiggling at everyone who came around. But smart dogs will sniff the hand of those they encounter before they let loose their full joy. And if they smell something that makes them suspicious, they know intuitively to hold back just a bit and wait for more information.

I was not so good at holding back, and I encountered a handful of individuals over the years who wanted to exploit my love but not return it, to take from me all that I would give and then demand more. And I willingly participated, which is something for me to own, and I do.

All kinds of dysfunctional behaviors masquerade as love, and we grab onto them with high hopes. No one is more confused than we are when we end up feeling stressed out, manipulated, and possibly abused. Part of learning how to properly love ourselves and others is learning to be discriminating, to watch for red flags, and to become able to identify exactly who and what we are facing. It may not always be love in other people. Sometimes it's addiction, sometimes it's lust, and sometimes it's possessive fear.

We can still be loving underneath, but in a calm and present way: steady, curious, and watchful. We must be cognizant of our responsibility to protect ourselves from harm. Perhaps the way to think about this is to imagine that at the end of our drawbridge there are two gates, an "in" gate and an "out" gate. We can keep our drawbridge down, but close either gate when necessary, or close either one partway. If we are unsure, we must proceed with caution. We, and we alone, are the gatekeepers of our loving energy, and how seriously we take this job will determine our sense of safety and well-being.

The neutral mindset we spoke about in chapter one is appropriate to consider in light of this discussion. We have a tendency to project positive or negative characteristics onto others based more on our internal state—our hopes and fears—than on the reality of who is actually in front of us. The point is to not jump to conclusions. If we find ourselves thinking we know who someone is and wanting to trust him or her implicitly, that is a red flag. Our internal voice, the same one that tells us when to stop eating, will guide us in this regard as well. So as we are learning to hear it, this is another place to listen for its wisdom. It will likely tell us to slow down and remain on guard, but we habitually blow right past it. We insist that we know better, but we generally pay a price, and often quite a steep one, for our insistence.

Appreciation Exercise:
Visualization for Healthy Boundaries

Visualizing the two following scenarios will help you appreciate your role as a loving protector of your beautiful self. In addition, you will come to understand the importance of observation and self-awareness in setting healthy boundaries. You will need a few minutes of quiet, uninterrupted time and an open mind.

1. Sit comfortably in an upright position so that you are relaxed, but not so comfortable that you might fall asleep.

2. Visualize a large swimming pool with lots of people in it. Everyone seems to be having fun. There is laughter and loud music playing and you feel drawn toward the activity. Two of your friends are waving at you to hurry up and come on over. And that's exactly what you do. You don't want to miss out.

3. As you approach the pool, a couple of guys in surfer trunks run over and grab you. They lift you off the ground and throw you in the deep end. They are laughing the whole time. You splash, startled, into the water, and sputter and choke. You're not a great swimmer. Disoriented, you flail about and doggy paddle over to the edge where you hold on and catch your breath before you climb out, awkwardly, and with a mixture of shame and relief. The individuals who threw you in are laughing at you. Feel what that feels like.

4. Open your eyes, stand up, and shake your arms and shoulders a few times before you sit back down and close your eyes again.

5. Visualize the same pool and the same scene, and feel the same attraction and the pull to be a part of it. Observe your friends waving at you to hurry up and wave back at them to acknowledge that you see them, but don't hurry. Stand back and watch for a minute. Observe that the pool has a shallow end and a deep end, and an ever-deepening slope from one to the other. Notice that there is a lot of activity at the deep end, and that a few guys in surf trunks are exceptionally rowdy and seem to be goading people on the sidelines to get wet. Watch as they pull an unsuspecting bystander who is completely clothed out of a chair and into the pool. Observe them laughing. Observe the shock and upset on the bystander's face as he emerges from the water.

6. Acknowledge silently to yourself that you are not a great swimmer and that you better stay away from the deep end and keep an eye out for the rowdy individuals. You don't want to be like the bystander who got thrown in.

7. As you approach the pool, you are aware of your friends urging you forward, and the slightly overwhelming chaos of the whole situation. You

proceed with care, fold your clothes neatly on a towel, leaving them a safe distance from the water's edge, and then enter the shallow end by using the steps. You lower yourself slowly to your neck, keeping your feet securely on the bottom of the pool the whole time, and smile at how refreshing the water feels.

8. Open your eyes and reflect: same situation, different approach. Consider which one feels more comfortable. Which one feels safer? In which of the two scenarios above are you better taking care of yourself? This is the one where your boundaries are intact.

Knowing that you can count on yourself to keep a lookout for danger and are able to set and maintain boundaries to protect yourself from harm will give you a sense of self-appreciation. Your safety is your responsibility, and learning to trust yourself to know what you are and are not willing to risk is empowering and affirming.

Review and Daily Action Plan

We must approach any new situation and any new people with as much caution as we approached the pool in the exercise above. Knowing who we are and what does and does not serve us is our ongoing job.

It is also our job to know when and where we are blocked to loving feelings, and to clear the blocks by being forgiving. We need to have the courage to be authentically ourselves; to continually grow love in our lives by being willing to communicate what's going on inside of us, and to express our appreciation and our compassion for the people and the things that populate our world. This is the way that we habituate ourselves to a life full of love. This is how we step up to experience the rewards of the real thing. It is not a game, not a farce, and not reserved for only a lucky few. Love is a way of being and a way of seeing that begins with willingness and ends with appreciation. It creates good feelings and makes for good living, and we can claim it for ourselves any time that we want.

1. Honestly evaluate how loving you are in all of your important relationships.

2. Identify your expectations of love versus the reality of your experience.

3. Be authentic.

4. Open to love as an ongoing strategy.

5. Grow compassion by recognizing the vulnerability in others.

6. Have the courage to recognize vulnerability as a strength.

7. Clear blocks through the process of forgiveness.

8. Grow loving energy in your life as a daily habit.

9. Establish and maintain healthy boundaries.

PART THREE

·····················

PRESENCE

"Wherever you are, be there totally."
—Eckhart Tolle

In this section of the book, our focus is on the way we experience time, and the importance of being grounded in the moment and aware of the concept of "presence." We consider the difference between doing and being, and discover that they are not mutually exclusive—that we can experience them both simultaneously, and that to do so is, in fact, a form of art.

In chapter five, "Awareness and the Purpose of Time," we examine how far we have traveled culturally from the cyclical, seasonal, sunup-to-sundown nature of time passing, to the modern fullness of multitasking and high-speed technology. We measure the way that our time is divided and weigh in on what's essential, and what is not. We consider why we may feel the necessity to distract ourselves, and face our fears and limiting beliefs surrounding the passage of time. The chapter ends with an exercise to help us show up fully for every moment of our lives.

In chapter six, "Turning Awareness into a Habit of Presence," we get quiet. And in the silence, we become mindful. We detoxify ourselves from technology and declutter our minds. We prioritize and organize with the goal of having ever-greater appreciation for each thing that we experience. We learn to say no and to set boundaries around the precious hours in our days as we come to understand that they are limited and that it is our spiritual responsibility to not overfill them. And then we commit to the ongoing practice of presence with a practical review.

CHAPTER FIVE

....

Awareness and the Purpose of Time

"We must run as fast as we can, just to stay in place."
—Lewis Carroll

Feeling like we can't keep up with the demands of our lives is a familiar concept to many of us. We have so much to do and so little time. We feel like we are catching up instead of keeping up, always harried no matter how well we plan, and constantly in a rush. And if this is not necessarily our problem, then maybe we feel the same kind of out-of-control frustration regarding the aging of our bodies and the incessant progress toward our ultimate demise.

Time seems to be in short supply, and we want more of it. There is simply not enough. And we are certain that if we had more time, then we would feel better. We would be happier, and we would have more satisfying lives. We blame technology and our jobs and all of the things that we have to do. There is, in fact, so much that we *have* to do that there doesn't seem to be any time left for what we *want* to do. We are victims of time, without choices, stuck on the merry-go-round of daily responsibility. Or we are victims of the aging process: infirm, immobile, and without purpose or direction. Either way, it's not much fun.

We long for rich experiences that will fulfill us and make us feel alive and happy, and yet, when given the opportunity for free and unencumbered hours, we laze around watching TV, drink too much and call it fun, or spend money we don't have on things that we don't need or on travel that stresses us out. And then it's back to work, or back to the same-old, whatever that may be, and we feel like we missed something. And maybe we did.

We live our lives waiting for something to happen that will change the way we feel—something that will make it all worth it. We wait for something, or someone, to save us from our internal angst and dissatisfaction. We wait, and we wait, and we wait. We get resentful from waiting. But that doesn't change the facts.

We live in a world that is rich with distractions, and it's easy for things of low importance to dominate our schedules. We are busy, but not necessarily productive. Our environment and the hours we keep drain our energy and we collapse into bed exhausted at night and then toss and turn because our minds are busy and will not let us sleep. We are out of balance and struggle though our days, with blips of enjoyment here and there, but largely burdened, and living for our "time off," such as it is. And then, at the other end of the extreme, are those of us who have too much time. In a nursing home, the clock seems almost arrested. Hours and days creep along, painfully slow and stagnant.

I have exaggerated, no doubt. We are not as bleak as all of this, really, but there is more truth here than we may care to admit. Most of us feel wronged one way or the other by the time we do or don't have, and readily complain about it. We either want more of it, or we want it to be different than it is.

The simple reality is that we have clock time for practical, daily matters, and a lifetime for our big-picture goals and the fulfillment of our purpose. And I would argue that most of us, without exception, believe that the two are mutually exclusive. We are either doing what we have to do—chores, errands, obligations, etc.— and taking care of them in our "clock time," or we are living our dreams in the special but limited way that we are able to do that.

We believe that our dreams are necessarily big deals—things we might put on a "bucket list" like traveling the world, skydiving, going on safari, or writing our life story. Dreams feel too important for the business of daily life. We save them for special times. And perhaps we even wait until we have earned the right to them. In our minds, we don't like to mix the mundane and the extraordinary. To us, it seems the right thing to do is to keep them forever separate.

But maybe there's a way to make our whole lives extraordinary. Maybe, in fact, our whole lives already are extraordinary, and we just don't realize it. Perhaps our life purpose happens as much in our small daily acts as it does in the satisfaction of our greatest hopes. And if we become willing to shift our perspective, perhaps we can transform the less-than-satisfying way that we currently relate to time and begin to experience every moment and every day as the exceptional experience that it actually is.

Sunup to sundown, and cyclically, is how we live. We revolve like the earth we inhabit. So part of being present and not worrying about the past or the future has to do with remembering this fact and limiting our concerns to the block of time we are in: preparing ourselves in the morning, reviewing our day at night, and enjoying the hours in between, making progress in small steps as we go.

We learn, in this way, what we can reasonably accomplish in each block of time, and what constitutes a good balance of work and pleasure, intensity and frivolity, physical and mental effort, alone time and social time. The challenge, for most of us, is that we are all out of whack and have no balance at all. We work too much, or sit too much, or have too little fun. And we have no real understanding that things could be different. Perhaps we even have the idea that life is supposed to be a test of some kind—a test of endurance, sacrifice, or difficulty.

We put off our relaxation and laughter and playfulness for semiannual vacations instead of making these things part of our daily fare. But I absolutely believe that it's possible to experience a mix of spirituality, productivity, movement, pleasure, love, compassion, intellectual stimulation, conversation, meditation, relaxation, emptiness, fullness, courage, and sleep all in the course of a single day. And that's the short list. We cage ourselves by making it only about one thing (or just a few things), and by driving our daily agendas like steam engines at full tilt.

But traveling at that speed, if we encounter unexpected roadblocks in the flow of our day, we easily lose our cool. We get angry and stress rises inside of us like a tornado. We spew it out into the space that we occupy and onto the people who are unfortunate enough to get in our way. We go on a tirade, righteously justified, of course, and miss seeing all of the small blessings that we trample over in our hostility and haste.

It doesn't have to be this way, not ever, and not for any of us. This kind of behavior is not what the spiritual journey is all about. It's about active and dynamic adjustment to the revolving currents of life, and enjoying each thing as it presents itself before us.

Honesty Exercise: How Do You Spend Your Time?

By honestly completing the exercise below, you will be able to see where you spend the majority of your time and properly acknowledge where you might be slightly, or severely, out of balance. You will need a pen or a pencil, your journal, and a few minutes of quiet, uninterrupted time.

Consider the list below, and next to each word and concept, put a plus, minus, or equal sign in order to indicate whether you want/need more (+) or less (−) of it in your life, or if you feel it's reasonably in balance (=).

_____ Work/ Career	_____ Community	_____ Structured Time
_____ Play/Fun/ Relaxation	_____ Solitude	_____ Unstructured Time
_____ Love/ Romance	_____ Exercise	_____ Education
_____ Friends	_____ Eating Mindfully	_____ Creativity
_____ Family	_____ Spirituality	_____ Travel

Once you have completed the list, take a few minutes to write in your journal, expanding on what you have marked off and expressing in your own words what you would like to see manifest differently in your life. Complete your journal entry with the statement, "I am willing to change."

EXAMPLE

– Work/Career	= Community	– Structured Time
+ Play/Fun/ Relaxation	= Solitude	+ Unstructured Time
+ Love/Romance	– Exercise	+ Education
= Friends	+ Eating Mindfully	+ Creativity
= Family	+ Spirituality	+ Travel

I feel fairly balanced in the way that I interact with people, whether they be friends, family, or the greater community at large, and fairly balanced in my alone time as well, but when it comes to romance and unstructured relaxation, I tend to be too practical and schedule-oriented to allow for much of it. There is a need in my life for more meandering and less demand: more downtime, creativity, and flow; less drive, rigor, and intensity; and more time to travel and explore, both the broad world and the depths of my own being. I trap myself in my own schedule by working extreme hours and believing that I am indispensable, and, being a personal trainer by trade, I overexercise on a daily basis as a part of that picture.

The general situation is too much work and not enough play. I am serious and overly productive. Some of that is a good thing, but too much keeps me off-balance and makes it seem as if I have something to prove, which I don't. By living with such an exaggerated sense of purpose, I unintentionally deny myself the freedom and the pleasure of slowing down and allowing my life to unfold. Sometimes it feels as if someone, or something, is in constant pursuit of me and trying to run me down, and all I can do is stay one step ahead. I know that there's a better way, and I want it. I am willing to change.

———

Self-reflection is an important tool for personal evolution. By thoughtfully considering the way that you are behaving in relation to time, as you have done above, you will have the beginning insight that you need to initiate change. By identifying where you may be out of balance, you can raise your awareness and make adjustments in your behavior that will allow you to experience more of what you want in your life.

How Attitude Affects Our Experience

Understanding where we are spending too much or not enough of our time is a useful exercise, but perhaps the real change that we need to make is more of an internal one. If we need more fun and play in our lives, then we can bring a greater sense of play to our work rather than change jobs or work less. We may need to adjust our thinking habits rather than physical ones because our attitude is ultimately what determines our experience, and not the other way around.

Plus, everything in life is an interrelated mix. We can set out to have "fun" and have no fun at all. It's not what we do with our time that dictates how we feel but how we feel that dictates our experience of time. It's impossible to separate life into clean and perfect categories. Everything bleeds into everything else.

And we have less control than we would like to believe. During any given day, our plans may be altered or derailed by circumstances we have no ability to affect. We frequently become subject to changes in our schedules that we have not chosen. So we need to carry the information from the last exercise with us on more of an internal plane than an external one.

From the journaling example above, if I need more meandering in my life and less demand and intensity, then that is an attitude I have to bring to everything. It's not enough to somehow try to schedule "meandering" into my day. I have to let go of my intense attitude and my rigor in regard to everything. If I don't want to feel as if I'm being chased, then I have to stop running as fast as I can, metaphorically speaking.

One of the reasons that we become so harried in life is because we go through the motions of activities without actually being present for them. Our minds are elsewhere as we drive to work, talk to our children, and sit down to eat. We race around, rigid and intense in the way we think about what has to be done. That's why it feels rigid and intense to do it. We have become thinking and doing machines and often completely miss out on the whole idea of being. Yet, if we were able to bring a bit of this being-ness to our time in the form of presence, I am certain that we would feel more balanced and more satisfied overall.

Doing and being need not be separate. They can both happen simultaneously. Learning to be present for every moment of our lives is a conscious skill, a form of art, a habit that we can develop, and one that will change everything for the better in our lives.

Awareness Exercise: Doing and Being Meditation

By washing your hands in the manner indicated, you will experience, and thereby understand, how a simple and ordinary activity can become a source of great pleasure and an extraordinary event. You will need a few uninterrupted minutes, a sink, a towel, and some soap.

1. Take a few deep breaths and make a conscious decision to bring your full awareness to the experience of washing your hands.

2. Turn on the water in the sink and listen to it running gently as you adjust the temperature to soothing warmth.

3. Wash your hands mindfully, paying attention to the warm, wet water on your skin, the smell and feel and lather of the soap, the rubbing together of your palms, and the sound sensations—all of it. Take your time, and really enjoy the process.

4. Continue the meditation as you dry your hands, feeling the texture of the towel against your fingers and skin, and then the dry, clean feeling.

5. Option: apply hand lotion in the same mindful manner.

Washing your hands as described above is a far different experience than performing the same action half-consciously with your mind racing ahead to all of the things that you have to do. We can learn to live our whole lives with this kind of present-moment awareness. It's a change in habit, a change in perspective, and a change in our level of intention, nothing more.

Time as a Gift

The time we have is a blessing. It is not a guarantee. And how we relate to it is our personal choice. We can savor it, begrudge it, or waste it. We can spend our time waiting for something better to come along, or we can glorify and appreciate each new day and every moment that transpires. We can choose to live in celebration, or in angst and regret.

Time is also relative. Einstein established that truth. If we are enjoying ourselves, time flows gracefully, and smoothly, without hiccups. And if we are miserable, it creeps and crawls. It hitches and hangs us up. An hour can feel like a minute or feel like forever. If we are doing something we want to do, time is a lot more pleasant than if we are doing something we have to do, and if we resist our experience, we suffer for it.

But if we're honest with ourselves, then we realize that we don't actually *have* to do anything. We only think we do. It feels almost instinctual to rail against this point. How can it be so? Clearly, we have to do this and we have to do that. We have to eat, sleep, bathe ourselves, work, and take care of all of the things that we take care of. No, we don't. Not any of it. Everything we do, we choose to do, even if that's not the story we tell ourselves.

Time is also less linear than we may think. In spite of our drive toward accomplishment and achievement, there is no absolute point of arrival, not even in death. Given the possibility of reincarnation, the evidence of near-death experiences, and the uncertainty of what comes next, the only thing we can really say is that time, as we know it, is experiential. It comes and goes, and then comes and goes again. It is circular, seasonal, and more like a spiral than a straight line. In the big picture, if we're honest, time must always remain a bit of a mystery.

In each individual moment, however, blessings abound; this is true no matter what. Our ongoing life circumstances may be full of emotional challenges—the suffering of loved ones, loss of income, sickness—but the moment is ripe with goodness, full of sensory pleasure and beauty if we will only pay attention enough to notice it. We can tune in to color and sound, the feeling of our breath in and out, the beating of our heart, the touch of our skin, our feet in our shoes, the warm sun, a gentle breeze, or a booming thunderstorm: whatever presents itself.

Multitasking, in this light, is a sham. It robs us of the pleasure we can get from experiencing one thing at a time fully. And experiencing one thing at a time fully is the art of good habits at its best. Present-moment awareness, as defined earlier, is a fundamental key to our long-term happiness.

But for most of us, these moments of presence are few and far between, and the majority of our time is spent in incessant thinking and unconscious doing. We think about the past or the future, who we're mad at, and how miserable we are. We do our daily duties mindlessly while complaining to ourselves inside our heads about everything. We are expert at being victims, and self-pity becomes a kind of "go-to" mindset. We lose our beautiful moments when we give in to our circling thoughts. We forget that time is a gift and become preoccupied with self-created problems while absolute satisfaction and everything we could ever hope for is in the simple experience of exactly what we are experiencing!

Why We're Not Present

To give ourselves some benefit of the doubt, it's assuredly difficult to have a quiet mind and a level head in our modern world, where everything is moving so quickly and demands for our energy, insight, and effort are voluminous. It's simpler, no doubt, to be fully present when we're sitting on a beach listening to the waves roll up the sand and recede than it is when our phones are ringing, the stack of paperwork on our desk is growing, our boss is banging on the door, and our partner is sick at home. We are pulled in multiple directions by our obligations as well as our desires.

The high-tech world in which we live is a busy place, and it's easy to be drawn off course. We can set out in the morning prepared to remain calm no matter what, with a meditation and some affirmations under our belts, and by lunchtime, be completely overwhelmed and crawling out of our skin with frustration. Intentions alone, and a positive mindset, will not save us. We have to practice presence, and keep on practicing it.

But this is difficult to do unless we organize and declutter our lives and learn how to be quiet from both an activity and a thinking perspective. It helps to create an environment that's conducive to presence by setting boundaries, not taking on more than we can reasonably handle, and accepting our limitations, which may be the most difficult task of all. We will address these issues one by one in the next chapter.

But for now, we need only understand that grounding ourselves in the chaotic rushing landscape of modern-day life is our personal responsibility and that things will go much better for us if we are willing to do the work required. Creating daily habits that support our intention to live mindfully and experience the fullness of every moment of our lives is worth the effort, and comes easier the more we do it. Over time, such habits take less and less of our intentional focus and give us more and more support.

But before we can take action to develop new habits—habits to help us keep our time clear of clutter, busy-ness, and too much all-around doing and thinking—it's important and valuable to understand clearly what is essential to us, and what simply is not.

Awareness Exercise: Discovering What Matters

In considering how you would change the speed and structure of your life if you were guaranteed more or less time to live, you come to understand what really matters. You will need a pen or a pencil, your journal, and a few minutes of quiet, uninterrupted time.

1. In your own words, answer the following two questions:

   - If you knew that you had only a short amount of time left to live (a year or less), what would you change in your life? What would you be sure to do, or to stop doing? Why?

   - And if you were guaranteed to live far beyond ordinary expectations, to say, 150, in good health, what would you change? What would you be sure to do or to stop doing? Why?

2. Using information from your answers to the questions above, list 3 to 5 things that you consider "essential" in your life. Decide what's most important.

+ If I had only a short amount of time to live, I would restructure my life. I would slow down and make sure to appreciate each day. I would continue to work, at least initially, but at a more enjoyable pace. And I would spend more time with my husband and children. A few long-dreamed-of vacations would become priorities, as would the writing of my memoir. I would choose all of my activities and energy expenditures with great care, and not be reckless. Mostly, I would live with care and awareness, so as to make each moment count.

+ If I had another hundred-plus years to live in guaranteed good health, I would also take more care about my choices, so as not to burn out. I would slow down and make sure that my work and time and energy were spent in as enjoyable a manner as possible. I would stop rushing, stop making excuses, and stop living in fear. I would enjoy my family, and enjoy doing less than I currently do on a daily basis. I would study more and write more and maybe go back to school—or maybe teach school. I would take more care maintaining my home, my car, my body, and my finances. I would take more care maintaining the overall quality of my life.

What's Essential in Both Cases:

1. Slowing down

2. Doing less

3. Choosing with care

Completing the exercise above as suggested should give you a clear understanding of what's most important to you in your life. You can use this information as motivation to reprioritize your schedule so that you are best honoring yourself.

Pleasure in the Mix

The point is, in either direction, why don't we do those things now? Why would the guarantee of more time or less time change anything? Are we living compromised lives based on outdated assumptions? Are we assuming that we will have time to straighten things out "down the road," or time for happiness "down the road"? Or, on the other hand, are we assuming that we have to get it all done right away because otherwise we won't be able to finish, so we better rush and hurry and no matter how fast we go we're not going fast enough? Are we afraid that we will run out of time?

It's nonsense, both ways. And yet, isn't this exactly how we live, alternating between these two states? It comes back to the concept of the present moment. All we really have, all we ever really have, is the moment that we occupy. In an instant—in any instant—some crazy shooter could come from out of nowhere and kill us, or we could die in a car crash, a mudslide, or a tree branch could fall and hit us on the head in such a way that our lives end instantly. These things happen all the time to all kinds of people who, like us, feel immune to these possibilities, feel certain of tomorrow and next year. But there is no such certainty for any of us. So "How important is it?" and "What really matters?" are important questions to keep in mind.

But this fatalistic view of life can make it all seem futile. Why work at all? Why bother with anything? And I would answer, because that is exactly where our joy lies. A rich and fulfilling life is a balanced life. It's one part duty and one part spontaneity, one part community and one part self. It's family and friendship, work and time off from working, spiritual and material. It is the honest enjoyment of each realm and every situation, and the overall experience of the mix.

All one thing or all another would be dull. Sometimes we try for that, but it doesn't satisfy. We need productivity. We need responsibility. These are not things we have to do with a sigh and a sense of burden. They fulfill us in the way that only they can. The pleasure comes from being fully conscious while we're doing them. The pleasure is in the experience of the moment, whatever the moment entails.

What Blocks Us?

One of the things that makes it difficult to experience the present moment exactly as it is, besides our endless and incessant thinking, is that we are wedded to specific expectations. We have plans for the day and plans for our lives. We decide what matters from an achievement perspective and set about making that happen. We lose sight of the path and the journey, and become all about the point of arrival. And we hang our hopes and our happiness on that distant point. We tell ourselves, "I will be happy when … (fill in the blank)." We're all familiar players at this game.

And when we get to the goal? When we arrive? We're still not happy. It's not what we expected. So we throw the line out again as we work toward the next thing, and the next. We don't understand and appreciate that what makes us happy ultimately is experiencing the present moment with all of its fullness right here and right now. There's no trick, no test to pass, and no great reward. There is the simple but profound gift of time, and our conscious ability to receive and appreciate that gift.

Another thing that blocks us is our inner critic. This is a dysfunctional manifestation of our helpful and trustworthy inner voice, and most of us have one. The inner critic not only conveys thinking, but judgment. It is the sound of "should." We hear, think, and believe that we should be doing this, that, and the other thing—anything other than what we're doing. We should be more productive, further along our career path, making more money, doing more volunteer work—whatever it may be.

Lack of stillness and lack of silence also block us. If we never slow down enough to stop spinning, then all we do is spin, like a spinning top. And there's no ability to be aware or careful when we're spinning.

We are also blocked by the distraction of technology, as well as our insecurities and fear: our powerful, overwhelming desire to control our lives and control outcomes, and control every detail of our situation. We become certain that if we don't control everything we can, we will somehow fall off the grid or cease to exist in any meaningful way. This is irrational, but such is the nature of fear.

And then, on some level, we may simply be blocked by our naïveté. We don't know that there's a better way, so we don't practice it. But by bringing higher awareness to our situation, and by reading this book, we do know. We know now. So let's find a way to move forward from this moment free from excuses.

Willingness Exercise: Letting Go of Blocks

By symbolically "washing away" the negativity associated with the concepts listed below, you will feel relieved and refreshed. The exercise requires a sink; shower or bathtub; soap; and a towel.

1. If you are right-handed, get your left forearm wet, and lather soap thickly from your elbow to your wrist. If you are left-handed, lather the right arm. You can do this mindfully, bringing full awareness to the water and soap like you did in the earlier "Doing and Being Meditation" on page 154.

2. Using your pointer finger, write the word "expectations" in the lather on your arm. It doesn't have to be perfect, just representative and symbolic.

3. Look at what you've written for a moment, and consider all the times you have said, "I will feel better when … I will be happy when … Everything will be okay when …" and become willing to let go of your expectations.

4. Let the water run across your arm and watch the word and the lather wash away.

5. Repeat steps 1 through 4 with the words below, considering the way each one negatively manifests in your life. Possible letting-go statements are listed beside each word for when you make the decision to let go.

   + SHOULD *(I release the energy of "should" in my life)*

   + RUSHING *(I let go of my need to rush)*

   + NOISE *(I let go of excess noise and welcome the peace and stillness of silence)*

   + FEAR *(I let go of my fear of the future)*

   + CONTROL *(I let go of my need to control every second of my time)*

6. Continue to let the water run across your arm, removing all remaining lather, and feel cleansed.

7. Use the towel to mindfully dry your arm.

The exercise described above is a demonstrative process for letting go of concepts that you may be negatively attached to, either knowingly or unknowingly. You could also write the words on a piece of paper and throw them in a hearth fire, or put them in a box and symbolically "turn them over" to God, or the Universe, or whatever you want the box to represent. Or you can create some other letting-go ritual of your choosing, which can become a useful, ongoing habit. In life we need to let go of all kinds of things, and then let go some more.

Regarding Habitual Lateness

Something else we need to let go of, if it's our issue, and let go of for good, is being late for everything. Lateness on occasion can't be helped, but lateness as a habit creates a problem in our lives. Over time, it can become a vicious cycle of unreliability, and consequently, does not support us in our desire to feel good about ourselves. To others, it may appear that we value our time more than theirs, which means being late attracts negative attention to us.

There are multiple reasons why we might be consistently late for things. Perhaps we overschedule ourselves and try to squeeze more things into our day than the day can hold. Like trying to pour a gallon of water into a quart-size bottle, it simply won't fit.

Or perhaps our habit of lateness is about something more emotional and deeper than that—low expectations of ourselves, or a punishing kind of self-fulfilling prophecy. We let other people down. They express their disappointment, and we feel like we have gotten what we deserve. This is a sad, but fixable, state of affairs.

Another reason for lateness is being a victim of time itself. We can get into a state where we hand over control of our time to others. We let them keep us on the phone long past a deadline that we have elsewhere, or we overstay at an appointment because we're uncomfortable setting a boundary and saying that we have to go.

The cure for all of these possibilities is no different than the cure for changing other habits that don't serve us. We honestly appraise our particular situation and admit to whatever imbalance exists, become willing to do the work to improve our condition, make a commitment to change, and then take action steps to manifest a different reality for ourselves. We try things; some of them will work and some won't. Any change is halting progress, and we might not get it absolutely right the first time, or even the tenth, but if we stay the course it does get better.

If we are challenged by being on time for things, an hourly planner might be a useful tool, as might the temporary support of an organizational coach. We can take a time-management course, or speak with a therapist if we think that will help. But the bottom line is that our well-being is ultimately our responsibility, and being habitually late does not support our well-being.

We can be compassionate with ourselves, but also real. It's possible to be disciplined, organized, and on time without losing our sense of spontaneity. Habitual lateness is not insurmountable. If we take ownership of our part in the cycle, we can step up and make the necessary changes in order to experience the results we desire. We may need outside help with this, but it can be done.

Time as It Is

The truth about time is that it's organic and beautiful. It is not something to fight, or something that is going to run out on us or chase us down. It's simply the cyclical nature of days and weeks and months and seasons.

We can be grateful for a fresh start every twenty-four hours, and grateful for the way time matures us—for smile lines around the eyes, and the calm that comes from a long life lived. We can be grateful that teenage years pass, for births of all kinds, and for the end of physical suffering in the peace of death. We can be grateful for the slow revelation of truth over time, the repetition of holidays and weather patterns, and the circling daily routine of good habits. We can be grateful for the closure of nightfall, and the waxing and waning moon, for mornings and afternoons, and for our ongoing personal evolution one day at a time.

Perhaps we have been wrestling with the pace of our lives. Perhaps we have felt time to be impossible to come to terms with, evasive and conniving, always eluding us. And yet, in some way, time has been carrying us the whole distance, and leading us forward, and giving us room to grow and to heal. Time, in its way, seems to know better than we do what we need and how long things take.

"All in good time," we live our lives, follow our dreams, and make our way. We are protected from too much change too fast by the very nature of our twenty-four-hour cycles. We can change in small bits and adjust here and there. We can grow goodness slowly and become solid, and more solid still, as the months and years advance.

Being aware of the goodness of time is a beginning, but awareness alone will not create meaningful change in our lives. We need to change our habits, and to do so, we need action, so that's what comes next. But as in the first two sections of the book, preparing for action requires that we become willing to engage, and willing to make the effort. We need to make a commitment and affirm to ourselves that we will do whatever it takes, follow suggestions as necessary, and consistently raise our awareness as a daily habit, so that we can experience the richness of time as the gift that it is.

Willingness Exercise: Committing to Change

By taking a vow that commits you to the positive experience of time, you are more likely to stay committed long-term. You will need a pen or a pencil, your journal, a few minutes of quiet, uninterrupted time, and some way of your choosing to ceremonialize your vow: a flower, a candle, a song, or stick of incense—be creative and use something that's meaningful to you.

If you choose to use your computer, iPad, or smartphone, use font style, colors, and available tools to formalize your written statement.

1. Create a sacred environment by lighting a candle, putting a flower in a vase, sitting in a special chair, or turning on some kind of music that is meaningful to you. It doesn't have to be complicated, only sincere.

2. Make a vow that commits you to an ongoing positive relationship with the natural cycles of time. Keep it simple. You can use one of the vows from the examples below or create your own. Write it down or type it, and then say it out loud. If you struggle with habitual lateness, incorporate your intention to be on time in the body of your vow.

3. Blow out the candle, or create a ceremonial closure of your choosing.

4. Commit your vow to memory.

5. Repeat it daily.

Examples

+ I vow to slow down and experience the beauty of time.

+ I vow to consistently practice present-moment awareness.

- I vow to appreciate each moment.

- I vow to enjoy the process of time.

- I vow to be prompt.

If you are sincere, this simple act of making a vow to yourself, and to time, can change your life experience profoundly. It grounds you in good intention, and is an important first step on the journey toward presence.

CHAPTER SIX

· · · · · · · · · · · · · · · · · · · ·

Turning Awareness into Presence as a Habit

"With the past, I have nothing to do;
nor with the future. I live now."
—Ralph Waldo Emerson

In the last chapter, I suggested that it's easier to be quiet internally, and mindful, if we're sitting on a beach listening to the waves roll in and out across the sand than it is to be mindful in the midst of a frenzy at work. Then, I further suggested that what we require to experience more presence in our lives—at work, at home, or anywhere—is an internal change, rather than an external one. We have to create the space for presence within us in order to experience it on the outside: as within, so without. This is a concept we've already touched upon. So what we're after, and what we want to learn, is how to carry the serenity of the beach and the waves to where it counts the most in terms of our life experience.

We have also established that practical matters relate closely to our experience of spiritual matters, and vice versa. They have a symbiotic relationship. And so, in an effort to increase our overall spiritual experience and to carry out our vow to engage in an ongoing positive relationship with time, let's direct our attention back to the practical.

Preparation and Organization

Our time is valuable, and through good organization, we can make the most of it. We waste precious hours dealing with messes we have either created by being sloppy or that we have failed to clean up. Preparation matters deeply, and so do neat drawers and closets, to-do lists, and pragmatic routines for managing mail, laundry, grocery shopping, exercise, and fun.

Our first mistake is to oversleep in the morning. It sets us up to go rushing through the day. We start off behind schedule and never catch up. Hitting the snooze button multiple times creates an illusion of luxury, when in fact, with every five minutes that we linger, we actually increase the necessity for frantic action once our feet hit the floor—that is, unless we build in a few snoozes to our schedule, and if that's the case we have to be diligent about not over-snoozing.

The point is to wake up and allow plenty of time to get ourselves together before we have to jump into action. This way, we set a relaxed and spacious tone for the day. And this is true no matter what time we have to start. A few extra minutes of sleep is not worth the difficult-to-overcome running-late feeling that travels with us if we rush out the door.

We need time to thoughtfully consider the day before us and prepare our hearts and minds for whatever may come, so that we can meet it with calm instead of panic. We need time to eat something, and perhaps do a few stretches or calisthenics to get our circulation going as well. Then we can travel to wherever we're off to without cutting it so close that we are stressed out on our way, and at least have a few moments to gather ourselves once we arrive before we are required to be *on*. It's almost like show business. We have to get ready backstage so that when we step into the light we leave our petty fears and mental obsessions behind and are completely and absolutely ready to go. That way, we can show up bright-eyed and crisp with a big smile, knowing that we have taken the time to care properly for ourselves, so we can now turn our full attention and compassion to the world at large. This we might call early morning preparation.

The same rules apply even if we don't have to leave the house. At some point in the day, life requires of us that we turn outward, perhaps in a text or e-mail, but outward nonetheless. But first, we must turn inward. This is where our grounding, our guidance, our peace of mind, and our sense of having plenty of time comes from.

Willingness Exercise: Technology Detox

By having a noise-free, technology-free, distraction-free period of time each day, you will support your need for silence and restoration. I suggest that this exercise become a part of your morning routine, but you can choose to do it at any time of day—whatever works best for you. This is meditation in action, which is essentially what present-moment awareness is all about. Consequently, all you need is willingness.

1. Make a decision to have a period of time in your day—at least 20 minutes, and hopefully longer—that is silent and technology-free: no phone, no computer, no radio, no television, no screen of any kind in front of you, and no noise. If it's convenient for you, this technology-free time can happen while you're driving in your car (be sure to turn off your GPS).

2. Understand that making this decision, and committing to it, is one way you can carry out the vow to become more conscious that you made in the last chapter.

3. During this allotted time, perform every action in the same manner in which you washed your hands previously. Experience doing and being at the same time. Go slowly and steadily, mindfully; pay attention to each moment. If you catch your mind racing off wildly, bring it back to the action at hand. Brush your

teeth. Get dressed. Make your coffee, smell it brewing, and sip it; prepare and eat your breakfast. Perform each action with attention and great care. Or if you are driving, simply drive. Listen to the sound of the road, breathe deeply, feeling your breath as it travels up and down your spine. Feel the seat beneath you, and the wheel in your hands. Watch your thoughts as they come up without attaching to them. Get to know the way your mind works in the silence of no-technology.

4. Make this a daily practice.

Creating a habit of silence as described above will expand your awareness, quiet your mind, and allow for the practice of mindfulness. It may well become a routine in your day that you look forward to and particularly enjoy because of the stillness and peace that it brings to your life.

Aligning with Our Natural Rhythms

Once we have done our morning preparation, we then have a handful of hours until lunch. Perhaps they are filled with projects and reports and business-at-hand. Perhaps they are overflowing with unfinished situations from the day before, or perhaps they are unstructured and we create our own momentum. All that depends on what we do, but for all of us, life is lived in cycles of time that are regulated by our meals and our sleeps. This is why we do ourselves a great disservice by skipping meals or staying up all night. Such behavior throws our natural rhythms way off.

We have recurring mornings, noons, and sunsets—recurring energy cycles and recurring currents of productivity and relaxation. The day ramps up as the light rises. Activity increases, and businesses open their doors. Things get done in the morning. It's a fresh start, and we all have fresh vision and momentum. And then, late morning, we start to get hungry, and the day takes on a bit of an edge until lunchtime, when there is a perpetual sigh of relief.

After lunch is a sense of temporary sleepiness. In Europe it's siesta-time. But in America, we push on, and continue to be productive. Afternoon productivity has a different energy than morning productivity, however, and is more steady and stalwart. It's "settled-in" productivity. We have adjusted to the day. And so we carry on until it's time to go home, or eat dinner, depending how late we work.

Evening energy is a whole different world again. It quiets down and empties out. We head home, tired. We regroup with our family and our pets. Maybe we take a walk or go for a jog to get some fresh air. We gather at the dinner table and share stories of our day, or maybe we live alone and check in with family and friends by phone and share stories that way, or maybe we settle down with a good book or our favorite television show.

And then, night closes us in. The darkness invites us to rest and restore ourselves. We sleep, and in our sleeping, heal. The hurts of the day dissolve. The urgencies disperse, and we are wrapped in silence and mystery until we wake again.

What I have described is the "standard" situation. Obviously, we all approach our days differently. Some of us are night owls who are most productive at 2:00 am, some of us work extreme hours and don't even take the time to stop for lunch or dinner, and some of us don't work at all. We structure our lives around our own unique kind of rhythm and routine. But no matter what our schedules look like, or how empty or busy they might be, we all have a rhythm. We rise and sleep and do what we do in a repetitive fashion: day in and day out, week in and week out, just like the sun and moon, light and darkness. Our rhythm sustains us. And we can find pleasure and experience enjoyment in it. We just have to learn how to be mindful enough to appreciate the cycle as it carries us around.

Appreciation Exercise:
Daily Practice for Observing Rhythms

Acknowledging what you love about the rhythm of your daily routines will infuse them with a certain sacredness and specialness, increase your gratitude for them, and help you stay centered and grounded as you go through the motions. The only tools you need for the exercise are the spiritual principles of awareness and appreciation.

In the "Growing Love" exercise, we identified and gave expression to all kinds of things that we love. In exercises from this chapter and the last one, we have practiced doing and being at the same time by being mindful and present while performing activities. Combining these exercises, bring awareness to each cycle and rhythm of your day as you experience it. These are your routines and your habits. Identify which ones you love—there are bound to be some—and give expression to your feelings.

EXAMPLE

+ I love putting on my socks and shoes in the morning because I always give myself a little foot massage while I'm at it, and the massage feels good.

+ I love watching the steam coming out of the teapot.

+ I love the first time I step outside in the morning and the way the air feels on my face.

+ I love starting down the road on my way to work.

+ I love the way I come alive as soon as I start moving.

+ I love sharing stories with my clients.

+ I love being silly and productive at the same time.

+ I love making people smile.

+ I love watching the trees and the birds while I eat my picnic lunches.

+ I love the physical exhaustion I feel driving home, and the quiet, peaceful ride.

- I love preparing dinner and
  listening to old country music.

- I love to sit in candlelight and talk
  and laugh after we're done eating.

- I love to work on my computer at night.

- I love stretching and prayers before bed.

- And I love cozying up with pillows
  and blankets as I settle in for the night.

Learning to be observant and to acknowledge and appreciate the little things about your routines and the rhythm of your days will increase your experience of joy in life. By making this an ongoing daily practice, you will become more and more proficient at recognizing the pleasure in all of your simple everyday cycles which, paradoxically, expands your sense of satisfaction, well-being, and happiness in the big picture as well.

Making Adjustments and Eliminating the Unnecessary

Bringing higher awareness to the pleasurable cycles of our days as described in the exercise above will also increase our awareness surrounding the parts of our schedules that we do not love. These may be things to do with work or community responsibility, family, friendships, or something else entirely. We may have a visceral distaste for our commute, our need to talk frequently on the phone, grocery shopping, or whatever it may be. It's important to identify these as well.

We no doubt resist these things, and our resistance to them creates tension and discomfort within us. They interfere with our pleasure and weigh us down. But maybe they are not as absolute as we might think. Perhaps, as suggested earlier, if we cannot change a situation, we can make internal adjustments and change the way we feel about it—a simple matter of shifting our perspective.

If something we are doing displeases us, we can either change what we're doing or how we're doing it—that's our basic choice. Anything other than that leaves us in displeasure and resistance, which sets us up in opposition to our very lives. We "stress out" about it. We get sore necks and sore backs and whatever other physical manifestations of our resistance may arise. We get heartburn and muscle cramps and headaches. So we can either eliminate irritating activities or experience them differently so that they no longer irritate us.

Although I'm certain that we feel on at least some level that everything we do has to be done exactly the way we are doing it, I'm willing to bet that may not necessarily be the case. Adjustments can always be made. For example, we don't have to respond to every e-mail and text the second we get it. To do so is disruptive and interferes with our ability to create flow and momentum. We get going, find a steady pace, and are "on a roll," so to speak; then our phone makes its incoming text sound and we stop what we're doing to check. It could be urgent. It could be important. And maybe it is, and maybe it's not. Maybe it's someone else's urgency, and they want to put it onto us. But whatever it is, we have allowed it to disrupt us. Our flow is gone, as is our momentum.

Making constant allowances for these digital disruptions, it becomes frustrating at best to accomplish and enjoy anything of substance or duration. In light of this fact, one of our decisions to change our daily habits might involve setting aside specific time in our schedules for checking e-mails and responding to texts, and stop allowing them to be an "on demand" activity. We can choose to make ourselves a little less accessible to the outside world, and the demands of whoever may call, text, or e-mail us at any time of the day or night. We can still be accessible, but more on our terms and at our convenience.

In this same way, regarding every aspect of our schedules and our lives, we have the power to make small adjustments of our choosing to improve the quality of our experience. We are not helpless victims of whatever may be thrown on our lap. It's up to us how we respond.

As a general rule, we have a tendency to inflate our importance in the scheme of things. We make bigger deals of our to-do lists and deadlines than is necessary. We "over-busy" ourselves and wear our busyness like a badge of honor. We feel self-important and enjoy a certain buzz and a rush from having ten things going on at once. But if we make things bigger than they are, we eventually become overwhelmed by them and end up crabby and burned out.

The Grand Canyon is an exquisite example of what can be accomplished with patience and small, consistent effort over time. For seventeen million years, the Colorado River has run its daily course, and doing so, it has carved out the canyon, eighteen miles across at its widest. For the same millions of years, tectonic plates have risen and fallen, causing volcanic eruptions and earthquakes, seismic activity that has established islands and craters all over the surface of the earth. The ocean has receded. And generations of people have been born, and died. Even the longest of our human lives is a mere blip on the page of history. So how important is it really whether we answer that text within five minutes of having received it, or whether we get our project done today or tomorrow or even next week?

It's within our power to re-order our agendas if we choose to. In terms of how we load our hours and what we take on, it's up to us to say how much is enough and how much is too much. Maybe we take on more than we have to and are unrealistic about our limitations. Perhaps we don't want to admit that we can't do everything and then some, so we make ourselves sick by never stopping and by never saying no.

We are the gatekeepers of our time. It is our responsibility to schedule ourselves and create routines that serve our highest good. No one else will do it for us. If we look to the world, the world will fill our every waking moment with have-tos and hurry-up-and-waits, with shoulds and favors, you name it. It is for us to make the most of our time.

If we can't take something else on in the course of our days because we are already maxed out well beyond reasonable limits, we need to say so. We benefit no one if we destroy our well-being and our peace of mind by overcommitting. We can drown under too many obligations, even though they may make us feel temporarily needed and indispensable. It is up to us to say no, and to say it without fear or guilt, to anything and everything that does not serve us.

Awareness Exercise:
Daily Checklist for Establishing Boundaries

By examining the choices we are making, both consciously and unconsciously, each day for a period of time, we will be able to see the reality of our patterns. This awareness will empower us to make the best possible choices for ourselves going forward. You will need a pen or a pencil, your journal, and a few minutes of quiet, uninterrupted time every evening for a week or so—as long as it's useful.

1. At the end of each day, make two columns in your journal—a "yes" column, and a "no" column, and then complete the exercise by listing the following terms under the correct columns for that day. In other words, if you found yourself rushing around in the morning,

then you would put "rushing" under the "yes" column. By doing so, you are acknowledging that even if you did not consciously make the decision to rush, you rushed anyway. On some unconscious level, you said "yes" to rushing. Our goal here is to bring awareness to what we are choosing each day, whether consciously or not. If one of the terms does not apply to you, then simply do not use it for your lists; if you want to add something, then by all means, do so.

Group 1

+ waking up grouchy

+ rushing

+ being frantic

+ multitasking

+ worrying

+ arriving late

+ feeling overwhelmed

+ irritated with delays

+ feeling like a victim

+ no time to exercise

+ other_____

Group 2

+ awaking refreshed

+ having enough time

+ being peaceful

+ enjoying the day

+ trusting the process

+ being on time

+ feeling relaxed

+ being at ease

+ feeling playful

+ making time to exercise

+ other_____

Group 3

+ oversleeping

+ feeling time dragging

+ being bored

+ not enough to do

+ wasting time

- being unproductive

- feeling blah

- being cynical

- feeling disinterested in life

- no desire to exercise

- other_____

Example: Day One

Yes

- rushing

- arriving late

- being frantic

- feeling overwhelmed

- worrying

- no desire to exercise

No

- being peaceful

- having enough time

- enjoying the day

- trusting the process

- being at ease

- feeling playful

2. After writing the first day's list, take a moment to reflect on the tone you are setting for your life with your unconscious choices. Are most of your "yes" items from the first, the third, or the second group, or is it an equal mix? In the example, the "yes" items have come mostly from the first grouping, which is indicative of someone who works too much. The third grouping lists behaviors on the other extreme, which could indicate a lack of motivation. What does your list indicate about you?

3. Make a decision to bring higher awareness to the way you experience time each day with the ongoing practice of this exercise. As you proceed, make your choices more conscious and steer them in the direction of the second grouping, instead of the first or third.

4. Appreciate positive changes as they appear on your daily list.

EXAMPLE: DAY 5

Yes

- having enough time

- being on time

+ trusting the process

+ being at ease

+ making time to exercise

+ other: *feeling in control of my time*

No

+ oversleeping

+ arriving late

+ multitasking

+ feeling overwhelmed

+ no time to exercise

+ feeling like a victim

We say yes and no to things every day with our actions, our behavior, and our thoughts, as well as our words, so the more aware we are of what we're choosing, the better choices we can make. It is our awareness that empowers us.

The Choice Is Ours

Let's turn for a moment to the results from the "How Do You Spend Your Time?" exercise from the last chapter (page 149). In the example, time was out of balance by being skewed toward too much work and not enough play—too much drive, rigor, and intensity, and not enough meandering and downtime. In order to change that, as was previously suggested, it's possible to shift our internal energies. We do not have to work less to create more balance, we can simply be less serious and rigorous in our approach to work. We can learn to relax in the midst of productivity. We can bring spaciousness to our mindset and peace to our routines.

Instead of being tense and driven and going at things in a kind of attack mode with a particular outcome in mind, we can create the energy within ourselves to experience each moment with curiosity instead of expectation. In this way, we can change how time feels to us as it's passing, and what we do loses some of its power to dictate our moods.

Nonetheless, some activities certainly lend themselves better than others to our personal enjoyment. Just as each of us feels pleasure moving physically in a unique way, we each enjoy different types of social time, creativity, work, and play. Some of us are naturally outdoorsmen, and some of us are naturally programming wizards, or financial analysts, or artists, or moms. Finding and honoring what we love to do is part of our personal, spiritual journey. We cannot force ourselves to be anything other than we are, and understanding clearly what motivates us only helps to empower our path.

Regarding all of the things that we long to do but don't think we have time for, once again, it may be our perception that is flawed—not our circumstance. We may think that we don't have time to meditate, to walk in nature, or to read what inspires us. We may feel that it's an impossibility to follow our dreams. Yet, it's entirely likely that we sit down in front of the television for two hours every evening and watch shows that either upset us in some way because of their violence or implications, or that don't mean anything at all. Watching television, in this case, is a choice that we make, and it fills up hours of our time that could be spent getting a master's degree online, or writing a book, or doing yoga. We have choices, and we make them: that's the point. And we have to take ownership of the consequences that result.

Our time may be filled with all kinds of habits that don't contribute in any way to our higher good or our soul satisfaction. If that's the case, no wonder we feel unfulfilled! We tend to take on more and more in an attempt to feel better, instead of decluttering our time to make room for what's really meaningful, and what matters most. It's up to us to say when enough is enough, but this is a challenge because "enough" is such a difficult concept for us to grasp, living in the "more-is-better" mindset that we do. We think that no matter what it is, it's never enough. But we can choose to see things differently.

Aging Gracefully

Whatever is in place in our lives is in place. No doubt, there's a mix of things we easily enjoy and others that require more effort to appreciate. As suggested, adjustments can be made. We can do less, approach what we do with a different attitude, slow down, change our routines, and make ongoing adjustments as they seem necessary and as they suit us.

But what may soothe us most as we travel down the road of time is to recognize our part in the greater scheme of things. As we are born and grow, and age and die, we are as intrinsically linked to the cycles of night and day and the years that pass as an oak tree. If we are planted in fertile soil and survive the storms that come and go, our roots deepen over time and we grow in stature. We become more solid and more respectable with every passing season, and ever-more capable of withstanding the weather. We become strong. We provide shade to others. From years of observation and experience, we acquire the wisdom of perspective. We no longer need to insist on ourselves and make a lot of noise.

In modern America, we have a tendency to disrespect the concept of growing old, and yet, it is a *growing* journey, not a diminishing one. We so highly value youth and physical beauty that we miss the beauty of wisdom and a life well-lived. We are so easily reckless when we are young, and so gullible and naive. Our priorities are misplaced, and our peers ever-ready to lead us astray. There are endless potential pitfalls and poor decisions that we have to make in order to evolve. But we have an opportunity to become graceful as we age, to become less frantic and more trusting in general, less flippant and insistent, and more stable and wise.

The experience of time is an immeasurable gift, and we miss it by thinking it has to be some certain way instead of just being what it is, which is perfect, balanced, and ever-evolving. We are an intrinsic part of nature's cycles, and our lives are an ongoing process. As we are able to take ownership of our proper place in the order of things, we will realize that time is not our enemy and that overfilling our schedules and living in a state of stress and frenzy is always our choice and never our obligation.

Appreciation Exercise: Self-Evolution Visualization

The act of visualizing your life on a continuum and imagining the corresponding feelings that come with every age makes you appreciate the passage of time and the evolutionary process of your life. You will need a few quiet minutes and an open mind.

Sit comfortably in an upright position so that you are relaxed, but not so comfortable that you might fall asleep.

1. Visualize yourself as a newborn baby. See yourself being held with love, being bathed and clothed, fed, and changed. Appreciate that you cannot speak, walk, or do much of anything for yourself. Feel what that feels like.

2. Now visualize yourself as a toddler just starting to walk and use words. You are wobbly and adorable, still helpless in many ways, but learning to be ever more self-sufficient. Feel what that feels like.

3. Visualize yourself at age five, eight, twelve, fifteen, eighteen, twenty, and on up to your

current age, whatever that may be, and feel
the corresponding feelings with each age.

4. Appreciate the blessings that come with
all of these ages, and appreciate the challenges
as well. Appreciate all that you have learned.

5. Visualize yourself at age 100, in good health,
surrounded by youngsters—maybe your children,
grandchildren, and great-grandchildren, or
maybe just friends. Feel what that feels like.

6. Sit quietly for a few minutes and appreciate the different
feelings of different ages and the experience of time in
this way. Put one hand across your heart and the other
hand on top of the first. Take a few deep breaths.

Visualizing the passage of years in this way creates a context
for wherever we may find ourselves on the timeline of our lives
and gives us a sense of appreciation for this incredible, evolutionary journey.

Review and Daily Action Plan

To create an ongoing habit of appreciation for the time that we
have, the most important thing for us to do is to raise our awareness. We need to learn how to pay attention to the experience of
life's little things as well as the big things, and feel grateful for the
natural rhythms of our lives. If we are honest about what we do,

and how we do it, and become willing to simplify our schedules and slow down, we can enjoy each moment and the process of our days. We can align ourselves with the flow of seasons and the natural unfolding of events without having to push and force our agendas. We can realize what's essential and what's not, and enjoy the simple art of doing and being at the same time.

1. Honestly evaluate how you spend your time and become willing to create more balance.

2. Learn the art of doing and being at the same time.

3. Slow down, do less, and choose with care.

4. Let go of useless habits.

5. Commit to enjoy the process of time.

6. Create a daily noise-free, technology-free, distraction-free zone.

7. Learn to love the natural rhythms of your daily routines.

8. Set boundaries with yes and no.

9. Be grateful for the journey of your life.

PART FOUR

. . . .

PROSPERITY

"One must learn, once and for all, to stop measuring
spiritual riches with a worldly yardstick."
—Paul Ferrini

Like the other sections of the book, this one is divided into two chapters. Here our focus is primarily on the spiritual principle of appreciation and the related concepts of abundance, purpose, discipline, and generosity. In the chapter entitled "Fear, Appreciation, and the Abundance Mindset," we examine the general tenets and disadvantages of consumerism and consider how we measure value in our lives. We determine whether our priorities are misplaced, and if so, where. And then, we establish the purpose that drives our existence, create a personal mission statement to ground us solidly in that truth, and make a commitment to the ongoing path.

In chapter eight, "Turning Appreciation into a Habit of Prosperity," we do the work. We purge our lives of material clutter, and then we form a habit of generosity. We learn to give. We give money, time, effort, love, whatever we have. We stop asking "What am I getting?" and start asking "What can I give?" instead. We begin to relate to gratitude as an action word and show our appreciation for all that we have in the way that we care for it. This applies to people as well, and to ourselves. And as we learn to appropriately value who we are and who others are, and the beauty and the mystery in all of us and in nature, we will become ever more conscious of the way that we behave toward and honor our world and those we share it with. And in valuing what's truly valuable, we will feel and enjoy the ongoing blessing of prosperity in our lives.

CHAPTER SEVEN

••••••••••••••••••••••••

Fear, Appreciation, and the Abundance Mindset

"It's good to have money and the things that money can buy,
but it's good, too, to check up once in a while and make sure
that you haven't lost the things that money can't buy."
—George Horace Lorimer

No matter how much money and how many material things
we have, many of us live with a certain insecurity regarding
our fiscal position in the world. We are fearful of not having
enough, or, if we already have enough, of not being able to hold
on to what we do have. Or maybe we're afraid of the way that
others might mishandle what is "ours." We tend to be possessive and defensive when it comes to the things that we own.

We equate success with material wealth and are afraid that we will never measure up. We are afraid of losing our jobs, of not being able to pay our bills, and of the fluctuations in the housing market, the stock market—not to mention our looming and overwhelming debt. We are afraid of not having the right stuff, the best stuff, or the latest and greatest stuff. We spend money we don't have on things that we don't need to "keep up." In all of these ways, and many others, we give money the power to determine our worth.

Modern culture is, for the most part, a consumer culture, and the more we have the better we must be, or so the thinking goes. This sets us up in a negative mindset where the ends justify the means—a mindset that validates the idea that as long as we are materially well-off, it doesn't matter what we do, or how we go about doing it. In this scenario, anything goes, so fear rules the day. If nothing is completely off-limits, and nothing is completely unthinkable, then slippery behavior can win, so to speak, and we expend lots of mental and emotional energy wondering how much we can get away with. We push the limits out further and further until they seem impossibly far out—buying things on credit would be a good example here—and then we worry that our limits are unsustainable and that they might collapse at any moment. And the truth is that they might.

Living beyond our means materially is an uncomfortable spiritual position to be in as well. We become controlled by our urges and our wants and our having to *have*. We think we are supposed to grab all that we can, and make that the agenda and the point. Imagine children around a piñata when the candy drops to the ground. They push each other and move lightning fast to scoop up as much as they can gather. Each of them wants to be the one who gets the most, because there is a limited supply.

This is the same kind of limited supply theory that engenders fear within us financially, as if there is only so much prosperity to be had. We better grab our fill, we think, or we'll end up with nothing. We look to our neighbors and our peers. We spy on them to see what they've got, and then we make sure that we have as much, or more. We try to guarantee our security this way and assure ourselves that happiness is the result of having and owning nice things. But nice things can't make us happy, not in a way that endures, and it can be distressing and stressful to discover that fact.

The original purpose of money and things was for exchange and survival, but we have turned them into something bigger, such that our modern pursuit of wealth and property threatens to overtake the living of our lives. In order to enjoy the blessing of real prosperity, we have to look at the way that financial fear and insecurity may be interfering with our well-being, and potentially disturbing our peace of mind.

Honesty Exercise: What Are You Afraid Of?

Doing this exercise will help you understand your financial insecurities, if you have any, and then give you an opportunity to consider how realistic your fears might, or might not, actually be. You will need a pen or a pencil and a few minutes of quiet, uninterrupted time.

1. Put a check next to every item on the list that applies to you.

_____I am afraid of not having enough.

_____I am afraid of losing my job.

_____I am afraid of losing my house.

_____I am afraid of not being able to pay my bills.

_____I am afraid of bankruptcy.

_____I am afraid of not being able to buy what I need.

_____I am afraid of having to live hand-to-mouth.

_____I am afraid of not ever being financially secure.

_____I am afraid of being destitute.

_____I am afraid of overspending.

_____I am afraid I will never be able to pay off my debt.

_____I am afraid of how I will survive financially once I retire.

_____I am afraid that the stock market will crash.

_____I am afraid of losing clients.

_____I am afraid of the financial implications
of getting a divorce.

_____I am afraid of being taken advantage of financially.

_____I am afraid that people only like me for my money.

_____I am afraid of having too much.

2. Review the items that you checked, and consider
each one individually. Ask yourself if your fear
is realistic, and if it's not, put a line through
the entire statement, effectively crossing it off.

3. If your fear *is* realistic, imagine it happening—
worst-case scenario—and think about how you
would handle it. Chances are, you would find a
way to survive, so what would you do? Remind
yourself that you are resourceful and that you have
managed to make it somehow or other financially
thus far in your life. Run through the scenario
and see whether you think you could find a way.
If so, put the letters "OK" next to your checkmark.

4. If there is something on the list you feel like you could *not* survive, put a star beside it. (Once this part of the exercise is complete, every item you checked should have an OK beside it, or a star, or be crossed out completely.)

5. Go back to the item/s that have stars, and create an affirmation for each one to counterbalance your seemingly insurmountable fear. Write it in your journal, commit it to memory, and repeat it regularly.

EXAMPLES

+ I am afraid of losing my house. (seemingly insurmountable fear)

+ I trust that I will always have a place to live. (affirmation)

+ I am afraid of being destitute. (seemingly insurmountable fear)

+ I am willing to believe that I will always be taken care of. (affirmation)

By consistently repeating a positive statement like the ones suggested above—one that affirms your trust and belief in abundance—you may discover that your fear slowly dissolves over time. And what seems impossible to face now may slowly lose its hold and its power over your energy and your mind.

Appreciation

Chances are that we already have everything we need. In fact, chances are we have way more than we need. The more that we have, the more time and effort and attention are required to effectively manage and maintain our situation. And the more that we have, the more our possessions come to control our lives. We lose our freedom to our things.

Perhaps we can make do with less and have more as a result. We don't need ten of everything—we may not even need one of everything. But we get so caught up in the feeling that whatever we own is never enough. This is part cultural and part personal, but it seems to reflect an overall state of restlessness and internal dissatisfaction. If we are constantly in pursuit of "more," then it's unlikely that we appreciate what is already ours.

Appreciation is a spiritual principle and one that can operate as a guide for our entire way of life. It is a recognition and acknowledgment of what we have to be grateful for. It focuses on what we are blessed with rather than what we lack. The opposite of a state of appreciation would be one where we take things for granted and feel entitled. From this perspective we deserve things because we work hard, because our lives are a chore, because our parents were less than perfect, or because we're having a bad day.

A sense of entitlement is unbecoming both externally and internally. It demands things, is dulled by excess, and spreads feelings of victimization through our insides like a swarm of bees. When we are entitled, we feel like everybody owes us something. It's the epitome of the what-am-I-getting-out-of-it mindset. There's no satisfaction in entitlement, only an unending need for more.

Appreciation, on the other hand, is being happy with whatever is offered. It understands that nothing is owed, nothing is particularly deserved, and that whatever comes to us can be construed as a gift. If we are appreciative, we can experience great pleasure in the smallest and simplest of things. While entitlement stands with arms crossed and a foot tapping impatiently, appreciation is blissfully free from any kind of expectations. Appreciation is being surprised and delighted with the ongoing experience of life itself, and whatever life serves up.

Most of us are probably appreciative and entitled by degrees, and it may be unrealistic to think that we can live in a state of perfect appreciation at all times. But it's something to aim for, and the more that we appreciate, the better we will feel. Our role and responsibility in this is to change our thinking and behavior around material things. And this, in turn, will change the way that we experience spiritual things as well. This is the path to prosperity.

Appreciation Exercise: Less Is More Visualization

The purpose of this exercise is to increase your understanding of the paradoxical but true axiom that less is more. You will need a chair and a few quiet, uninterrupted moments.

1. Sit comfortably, but with good posture, and close your eyes. Take a few long, slow breaths.

2. Visualize a shelf display in a boutique store in an upscale neighborhood. See that the shelf is lined with black velvet and that the surface of it is jam-packed with tiny, decorative boxes. There are so many of them that it's hard to distinguish one from another. You like the idea of them, and look more closely. You need a birthday present for your friend and think she might like one of these boxes. Visualize yourself picking one up and turning it over to see how much it costs. The marked price seems high to you. You have made an assumption that these are simple and inexpensive trinket boxes because of the way they are displayed, and yet, the price would indicate otherwise. You can't wrap your head around it, and you can't pick one anyway. There are too many to choose from. Visualize yourself feeling frustrated as you walk away, and not giving the boxes another thought.

3. Visualize the same shelf display in the same store, but this time, with only three of the tiny decorative boxes on the black velvet backing. Each box stands out and you see that they are beautiful. You lean in for a closer look. The work is delicate and intricate, and they seem hand-painted and are inlaid with crystal chips. You

think your friend might like one and it's her birthday in a few days. Visualize yourself carefully picking up the one on the left—your favorite—to look on the bottom for a price. It doesn't seem like enough for the workmanship involved. Visualize yourself turning the box over in your hands and looking at it closely, appreciating all of the detail. You're not entirely sure about it as a gift, so you make the decision not to buy it, but as you walk away and move on through the store, the memory of seeing it and touching it lingers with you, and you feel a distinguishable sense of appreciation for whoever made that beautiful box.

4. Open your eyes and take a few deep breaths. Thoughtfully consider that the boxes in each scenario were identical, and that the only difference was that there were more of them in scenario number one. In this example, greater value was assigned to the boxes, and greater appreciation rendered, when there were fewer boxes on the shelf.

5. Using this visualization exercise as your guide, think of a real-life example where this same principle is at work. Some ideas might be your closet, your pantry, your desk, or your garage.

The lesson here, of course, is that less is more. It's hard to properly appreciate what we have when it's all crowded together and jumbled up. So keeping every aspect of our lives simple and our spaces clear of clutter is a gift that we can give to ourselves.

Measuring Values and the Principle of Abundance

In our material world, it's easy to lose sight of the real value of things. We become so externally focused that we fail to connect with the richness that lies within us. We forget about the immeasurable value of love and forgiveness, patience and present-moment awareness, courage and hope. And having become habituated to measuring the value of things by the cost, we fail to see and acknowledge the beauty of the earth itself, and the people and animals and plants that populate it.

From birth to death, ours is a miraculous experience. We have been given the gift of language and self-expression, laughter and tears. We see. We hear. We touch and feel. We have a heart that beats tirelessly and a mind that reasons and thinks. We create life, we raise children, and we grow old—and are blessed along the entire journey. We live in the presence of the sky and the earth. We experience sunshine and moonlight, rain and snow. This is abundance! It's simple, yet profound. And yet, distractible as we are, we miss it. We go our whole lives looking outward, looking to things and money for satisfaction. We look for wealth where we cannot find it.

Abundance knows that we are rich and prosperous with or without material goods. We can enjoy them, but they are not a requirement for our happiness. Abundance is an attitude, not the result of some particular standing in the world. It is authentic: the honest admission of what really matters and what has the greatest value, and the reality that we are already and absolutely in possession of these things.

Appreciation Exercise: Understanding Values

This exercise is designed to make you aware of the difference between material wealth and abundance. All you need is willingness and a few minutes of quiet, uninterrupted time. Consider these questions, and answer them honestly for yourself:

+ Would you trade your eyesight for a million dollars?

+ Why, or why not?

Take note of how long it took you to answer the first question. Did you have to deliberate and weigh the pros and cons, or were you able to answer the question immediately, with no doubt whatsoever?

Chances are that you would not trade your eyesight for a million dollars, a billion dollars, or any amount. And chances are that you didn't have to do a whole lot of pondering to decide what your answer would be. We don't generally think of our eyesight as something that's "for sale," and if we try to think of it that way, it's disconcerting. How can we possibly put a price tag on our ability to see? We can't. That's the point.

Beyond the Material

Our eyesight, like our ability to breathe, speak, hear, and touch, is something that we take for granted. All of our senses are useful adjuncts to having a body, but we don't generally think of them much beyond that. We take them for granted, that is, until we are asked to give them up. Then we realize their value.

As human beings, we have the ability to bring conscious awareness to ourselves and to our life circumstances. We have the ability to be *self*-conscious. As such, we can color our perception by twisting it any way we choose with our thinking. We can make it all rainbows or paint it black. Unless we learn to quiet our minds, we have endless running commentaries going on in our heads that disrupt and distort reality.

Abundance is learning to quiet this mental noise and to simply become conscious of the gift of the moment and all of the factors that contribute to that gift: our physical senses and what they are experiencing, the activity around us in our current environment, and features of the natural world like light, temperature, tree leaves, and birdsong. This is essentially the practice of presence, as we have already described it. The difference, with abundance, is that beyond the experience of the moment, there is a built-in experiential appreciation for every single element of it. It's not that we are judging the situation or thinking about it as being positive or beautiful or special or whatever, but that we are actually experiencing it that way. There is joy in our experience—not manufactured, thought-created joy—but the pure and essential joy of being. Becoming conscious of this primal joy in our experience of life itself, with all of its attendant wonders, is one part of the experience of abundance.

The Big Picture

Another part of the abundance-experience is related to our life purpose. From a doing perspective, we are not here exclusively to make a fortune or to sit around. There's something bigger and deeper for us connected to our energy and our spirit; something beyond money, beyond materialism, and beyond what we can see that is the reason for our being here at all.

Ultimately, we are spiritual beings, and as such, we have to learn to live by spiritual principles such as patience, tolerance, forgiveness, acceptance, gratitude, and love. These, and others like them, are values and guideposts to help us navigate our path, and they give us a sense of purpose. We are here to make the world a better place; to do good, to be kind, and to express our love.

Lacking this spirit-connected sense of meaningful purpose, we lack abundance. Living aimlessly with no guiding light, we are empty. Similarly, failing to understand cause and effect and failing to take responsibility for our spiritual well-being due to a preoccupation with material wealth, we may succeed on the material plane but feel only minimal satisfaction for that accomplishment.

We have to find a way to coordinate our material purpose (what we do) with our spiritual purpose (who we are).

In this way, our *life* purpose is tied in to our productivity, to what we produce and how we produce it in the physical realm. Which is not to say that we have to do work that is directly and obviously spiritual, not at all. We are responsible for bringing the spirituality to our effort. By being aware of how our work connects us to humanity at large, and how it serves others, we can make the most mundane jobs deeply meaningful. If we are washing dishes, we are bringing our energy to the plates and pots and silverware that others will eat off of, and as such, we have an important role to play. Our work affects others no matter what we do. If we try to make it about ourselves exclusively, or only about making money, we are missing the point, and we will miss the feeling of fulfillment as well.

Let's take the job of financial analyst or stockbroker as an example. If such an individual steers his clients toward the stocks that he knows will make him the largest commission regardless of the clients' particular inclinations and expressed desires, he will likely make a lot of money. And perhaps his clients will make money in the process as well. But he will nonetheless have dishonored them and dishonored himself. It is his moral obligation, and the spiritual purpose of his work, to share his expertise, give them choices, and listen to their feedback, thereby respecting them as individuals. He serves no one by simply pushing his personal agenda without consideration for their feelings.

An important part of our life purpose has to do with the way that we relate to others. We are social beings and live in communities. We cannot be rude and careless without paying a high price. We can pretend that we don't need other people and make it our mission to isolate ourselves from the world, and we can succeed in this to a certain degree, but we suffer for it. We are meant to interact. We are meant to exchange ideas, feelings, and experiences with each other. That's how we learn and how we give back. We all have something to offer and something to receive. In this way, not one of us is better than the other. We are connected by the fact of our being human.

We also have a self-honoring purpose in life. We are meant to take care of our bodies, our feelings, and our spiritual evolution. We have a role in our own education. It's up to us to do the footwork and follow our calling, and it's up to us to self-reflect. We must be active participants in our lives. We cannot sit back and hold back and expect our dreams and our happiness to fall in our laps. We have to do our part.

So what we do and how we do it, the way that we relate to others, the way that we honor ourselves, and our active participation in showing up for life are all contributing factors to our ultimate purpose, and our sense of abundance. But it's easy to lose sight of these things in our busy and chaotic world. We can be pushed and pulled off course in all manner of unhelpful directions. Because of this, a personal mission statement that clearly articulates our life purpose is a useful grounding tool. Such a statement can guide us in making decisions and keep us on track. It needn't be complicated, complex, or overthought.

Honesty Exercise: Creating a Mission Statement

In this exercise, you will clarify your life purpose by creating a Personal Mission Statement. You will need a pen or a pencil, your journal, and the patience to thoroughly work this process. Keep in mind, as you proceed, that the point of this statement is to capture the essence of your life philosophy and your life work. Whether the final statement is a complete sentence, an infinitive phrase, or a few choice words doesn't matter. What matters is that it speaks to you, translates easily to others, and succinctly captures the point.

1. Gather information. Write down the answers to the following questions in your journal:

   + What is most important to me? What matters most in my life?

   + What do I stand for?

   + What do I do for work and how do I do it? What are my goals?

   + Whom do I serve?

2. Write a few sentences or statements to summarize the information that you gathered above.

3. Reduce and simplify what you've written, fine-tuning it to capture the essence of what you are trying to say. Make each word count, and make what you've written work for you.

4. Commit your mission statement to memory, and let it guide your path.

EXAMPLES

+ My goal is to live with grace and to be of service, to have fun and be effective, to carry enthusiasm wherever I go, and to be kind and loving with all those I encounter.

+ I am dedicated to helping those less fortunate.

+ My purpose is to provide for my family and be a loving member of the human race.

+ I am committed to being honest and kind while still maximizing my material potential, and helping others to do the same.

+ I respect the environment in which I live.

+ To work in partnership with others and inspire health and well-being in the senior population.

+ Leading by example.

A mission statement is a guiding principle. It helps us to make a decision when we are faced with any and every choice. We know our purpose and what we are all about, and consequently, we are able to consciously and consistently keep our forward momentum in alignment with our intended perspective, our vision, and our point of view.

Discipline and Commitment

It's easy to nod our heads and agree with things in theory and to intellectually appreciate what's important and even to take some kind of intellectual ownership of our role in the process of our lives. But it's another thing entirely to maintain self-discipline and stay committed to the path of well-being. This is the art of good habits. If we repeat the right action enough times, it becomes instinctual, but at first it is all about paying attention and our willingness to do the work. Stops and starts and halfhearted attempts will give us limited results at best.

The abundance mindset is a choice. It's a choice to live by spiritual principles and in integrity with ourselves. It's also a choice to open ourselves to the experience of the moment, the joy of being, and all of the gifts and blessings that we already possess. The consequence of choosing abundance is a condition of thriving.

But if we want to thrive long-term, and not in little bursts, we have to solidly establish a habit of choosing abundance every day of our lives, without reluctance. This means that we have to practice catching ourselves slipping into bitterness and fear. We have to learn to watch our minds for negative judgment, sour grapes, the justification of seedy behaviors, and physical and emotional abuse of ourselves or others. And we have to be vigilant about it. When we discover ourselves in the act, so to speak, we have to be willing to make the choices that will lead us back to abundance and back into alignment with our personal mission statement and our spiritual values. This is similar to the "Catching Yourself" exercise from chapter four.

Getting off track is easy, and getting back on track is relatively easy as well. What is difficult, and what requires all of our discipline, especially in the beginning, is to stay on track. It requires steady and consistent evaluation and adjustment; self-questioning, self-honesty, and self-awareness. We have to bring attention to our feelings of entitlement and resentment. We have to hear our own whining and shut it down.

Initially, as we change any habit of thinking or behavior, it seems like a whole lot of hard work. And it's our instinctual, default position when the going gets tough to give up on the process and return to what we know, where our results may be mediocre, but the expectations are clear.

We may read a book full of good ideas and truths that will help us change our lives for the better if we implement them fully. But once we're finished reading and have put the book down, the follow-through is up to us. That's where the rubber meets the road, and we have to summon up our inner drive. It's up to us to do the daily work. And if we do it steadily for long enough it will become easier and easier, so that eventually it will become second nature and we hardly have to think about it at all. But we still have to do it, because doing it is what gives us results.

Active and willing participation is our part in the satisfaction of our life experience, and it is a daily responsibility. And though there is effort involved, the work itself brings us pleasure. It is designed to make us feel good. So often, we approach life-improving propositions with a sigh and a kind of put-upon resignation. We agree to do what's suggested, but not with excitement. And yet, it's for our own highest good!

We need to find the inner motivation to help ourselves and do what we need to do in order to feel the way that we want to feel: satisfied, blissful, and enthusiastic about our lives. We have to commit to the path. We have to engage ourselves fully. We can experience radiant abundance and prosperity in our lives, no matter what our economic condition might be, but we have to commit to our part of the work, and then honor our commitment. It's a worthwhile adventure. What could matter more?

Willingness Exercise: Committing to Abundance

Performing this exercise as suggested will establish your commitment to the abundance mindset and the experience of prosperity solidly within you. You will need a few seconds each day to state the affirmation.

1. Read the following statement to yourself silently or out loud: "I am committed to experiencing abundance and prosperity in my life."

2. Memorize the statement.

3. Repeat it to yourself every day, at least once, or more than once if you feel inspired to do so, and make it a daily habit.

This is a form of self-programming. By stating our clear intention and using the tool of repetition, we can watch our intended reality begin to manifest in our lives. But it's only a beginning. Intention will only take us so far. We have to get into action to see it fully play out.

CHAPTER EIGHT

• •

Turning Appreciation Into Prosperity as a Habit

"We can only be said to be alive in those moments
when our hearts are conscious of our blessings."
—Thornton Wilder

A theoretical understanding of the abundance mindset is useful, but it is not enough to create meaningful change in our lives. We need to take practical action steps if we want to measurably increase the experiential level of prosperity that we feel.

First and foremost, we can purge our lives of material excess and physical clutter, and get in the habit of keeping them clear. Walking around our houses, we are likely to find all kinds of unnecessary stuff: overflowing drawers and catch-all closets; cabinets full of we don't even know what; and shoes, clothes, and linens that we haven't used in years. Things pile up. Stacks of paperwork, old catalogs, and newspapers clutter our tabletops. They may be orderly stacks, but they are nonetheless cluttering our space.

We have a tendency to save things for future use. If there's any possibility that we might need or enjoy something down the line, we are unwilling to let it go. And so we hold on, though there may be no reasonable purpose in our present situation: magazines that we would like to read if we ever get the time; pants and shirts that are too small, too big, or out of style but that we like anyway and hold on to for posterity's sake; and endless books, knick-knacks, cassette tapes (they may become collector's items someday!), out-of-date costume jewelry, broken tools, gadgets of all kinds, and children's toys.

We would sooner allow things that we are sentimental about or that we might need someday to jam up the energy of our lives than face the possibility of regret were we to give them away. And yet, by maintaining them in our homes, we rob ourselves of the feeling of cleanliness and spaciousness that's possible in an environment cleansed of excess.

Consider the visualization exercise from the last chapter with the ornamental boxes. We felt better about them, and felt they had more value, when there were only three of them. Less was more. And it is no different in our lives and in our homes. If we have more than we need or than we can appreciate, our sense of well-being is diminished. We become overwhelmed by the sheer volume of our stuff instead of being delighted by it.

And from a metaphysical perspective as well, too many things all cluttered and stacked together can trap the flow of energy and create stagnant pools of blocked creativity. Having overfull drawers get stuck every time we open them, lost mail in piles of junk paper, and disorganized cabinets and closets everywhere we turn leads to frustration, irritation, stress, and dis-ease—all self-perpetuated.

If we create a home environment where everything we own is essential, either because we love it or because it serves a particular purpose, then we will feel more appreciation for our home. If we pare down our closets, we will take better care of our clothes; if we eliminate clutter in our kitchens, we will increase our joy of cooking; and if we get rid of nonessential files and old papers, we will be less resistant to office work.

Awareness and Willingness Exercise:
Identifying and Eliminating Physical Clutter

This exercise will help you learn to see what's cluttered and disorganized in the physical spaces that you occupy, give you a system to clear the clutter, and a maintenance plan to keep it clear. You will need a pen or pencil and your journal, courage, willingness, patience, and follow-through. This is an ongoing, lifelong process, and though it may seem a bit overwhelming at first, you will get better at it the more you do it. And the results are well worth the effort.

Still, it's a big job, and as such, you may feel your resistance rising up even contemplating the idea. Using the guidelines provided here, I encourage you to trust the process. Start as small as you need to and build confidence and momentum as you go. And feel free to modify the approach in any way that feels right to you. What's provided here is meant to serve as a helpful example. These are not hard-and-fast rules.

The best approach for you may be to start by taking fifteen minutes to clean out a single drawer in your bathroom one weekend afternoon, or just throw away accumulated trash in your car. A "master list" as described on the next page may feel like too much to you. If that's the case, honor your feelings. In much the same way we described the "Learning to STOP" phenomenon in chapter two, it's important to address the most obvious clutter first. If things fall out every time you open a certain cabinet in your kitchen, or you take note of the disorder within and think, "I really need to straighten this up," that's the place to begin. Ultimately, the point is to use the steps below to guide you, but not to limit you. This is your process. I encourage you to make adjustments as necessary. Have your journal ready so that you can take notes and create helpful reminders for yourself as you proceed.

CLEAN-UP

1. Identify! Starting with the places where you spend the most time—your office, car, kitchen, bedroom, etc.—and then expanding outward to your entire home

environment as time permits, identify items that no longer suit your taste, bring up negative emotion, create a feeling of disorganization, or are in disrepair. Make a mental note of these things and create an accompanying master list in your journal. This will be a kind of ongoing, working to-do list. Cross off items as you address them, and add to the list anytime you see something additional.

As mentioned, if the idea of a "master list" is too overwhelming, then start with just one room, one section of a room, or whatever makes sense to you. You could approach closets first, or drawers, cabinets, or your desk. The point is to simply begin by raising your awareness and noticing what's cluttered, and what you own that doesn't please you anymore.

2. Donate! Recycle or throw away what is beyond redemption, and give away what has lost its purpose for you personally, but still has value. Locate a Salvation Army, thrift store, or other charity service near you that accepts donations. Get the address of a drop-off location and drop-off hours, and establish a connection with a service that will pick things up from your home as well.

3. Sell! Consider the option to open an account on eBay or Craigslist for items you would rather sell than donate or find a service that will do this for you.

This cleansing and decluttering process can be time-consuming, and requires effort, which may be why we often choose to turn a blind eye rather than address it. It's important to keep things bite-sized, or otherwise manageable, so that you don't feel overwhelmed. Consequently, it's helpful to consider in advance when you can willingly make time for this process in your schedule. Perhaps you can dedicate an hour or so on Saturday mornings, fifteen minutes every evening after dinner, or a half hour once a week. Or if you prefer to take an entire day or a weekend every few months or once a quarter, or you can even let your decluttering schedule revolve around the set-up or clean-up of holidays. It doesn't matter when you address your cluttered spaces, only that you do.

Some jobs may be too large for you to complete on your own. You may need friends or a hired hand, or a professional organizational service to assist. Do what you can, and get help when you need it. But don't stop the work!

It can be challenging to know what to let go of and what to keep. We can err on the side of being too sentimental and keeping too much, or recklessly getting rid of things and feeling later regret. When faced with uncertainty, it's useful to consider what emotion comes up in regard to the item in question, and whether we want to promote or diminish that emotion in our lives. Our Mission Statement can help us in this process.

As a general rule, if you are on the fence about certain things, it's probably best to keep them. You can store them in a temporary, revisit-in-six-months bin. But if you are feeling this way about *everything*, you may need to involve a friend to help you let go.

Taking pictures of things as you release them may be helpful to you in this process as well. That way, you still have a record of meaningful items, but they no longer take up physical space. Considering how others may benefit and enjoy something you have enjoyed may also be helpful. If you give away something you have loved, it makes you feel good to think that someone else may learn to love it as well. Plus, it's far better from an energetic perspective to have things in circulation than packed away in boxes.

The Clean-Up part of this process is quite an undertaking, so be patient with yourself as you steadily work your way through it. Happily, though, once you have done the work, it's done. Then it becomes a simple matter of maintenance, which, by creating helpful habits, is fairly easy to sustain.

Follow-Up Maintenance

1. Create new ways to organize. When everything has a place, it's easier to keep things tidy. The Container Store and ideas on Pinterest can become invaluable to you during this part of the process. Having a hanging hook for your keys right inside the door, bins for mail, racks for shoes, baskets for dirty clothes, and all kinds of things along these lines can help keep your environment clutter-free. Have fun with this and use the space you

have to create clean efficiency and organization that makes sense for your particular location and situation.

2. Keep a tab on your physical spaces regularly and keep them clear. You might set a time each day—perhaps in the evening before bed—or a time of week—maybe Sunday afternoons—to go from room to room, picking up and reorganizing what's out of place.

3. If you notice drawers and closets start to fill up or become messy, a new organization method may be needed. Make adjustments as necessary to keep clutter and disorder from accumulating.

4. Keep a "donate" bin in a convenient area so you have a place to gather things you decide to let go of. This will ensure that items won't have a chance to build up as clutter and keeps the concept of letting go and giving to others at the forefront of your mind as well.

5. Recycle and dispose of unnecessary paperwork and junk mail on a regular basis.

6. Pause before purchasing anything new. Ask yourself, "Do I love it? Is it essential?" and if the answer is not yes to either question, walk away.

This can all be challenging work. The things we keep around us act as containers for emotion, so clearing physical things away can take time to process. But it is a practice that, in the end, becomes freeing and opens up physical, mental, and emotional room to receive something new. By identifying and eliminating clutter in your personal space, you will be able to better appreciate what you have and enjoy the satisfying feeling of less being more.

The Benefits of Generosity

In addition to the obvious benefit that we experience as the result of clearing our space and decluttering our physical environment, by giving some of our possessions away, we get the added benefit of being generous. What we no longer need or appreciate may be just what someone else has been looking for.

But on a deeper and more intentional level, the spiritual principle of generosity is directly and inextricably linked to prosperity. The basic desire to give to others is rooted in the understanding that we have more than enough. We have been blessed so generously that it follows naturally to share our wealth with others. And this is not strictly material wealth, but wealth of spirit, wealth of intellect, wealth of appreciation, intuition, inspiration, and the like.

In this case, we give what we have to give. We give our attention and our insight, our skills and our thoughtful consideration. We give sincere compliments, compassion, and love. We give our time, effort, vision, strength, and heart. We are team players and contribute whatever we can to the greater good. When living in the energy of this expansive generosity, we feel a part of people's lives. They are grateful for our generosity, and they say so. Consequently, we feel appreciated, needed, and encouraged to give more. And so we do, and the happy spiral carries us upward.

If, on the other hand, we believe that we don't have enough in life, whatever that may mean to us in particular, then it's unlikely that we will feel generous at all. We will be more likely to hold on to what we have and be somewhat miserly about it, feeling suspicious of others in case they have a desire to take it away. In this case, we are reticent to share anything with anyone and prefer to keep to ourselves, because that's where we feel the safest. Any kind of loving exchange or human connection is hampered by this point of view, and the result is isolation, separation, and more of our not-having-enough feelings. It's a cycle that feeds on itself and in this case, spirals us further and further into despair. We feel that no one can be trusted and we grab for more of anything and everything in order to get what we feel we need. We are not generous with others, and so very few people are generous with us.

But what we actually need, as human beings, is a loving and generous exchange with other people. We need to share the wealth of our beautiful selves. And if we have material abundance to share with others as well, all the better, but that's not a requirement. The only requirement for the experience of prosperity is a generous attitude. Everything follows from that.

The expression that "we get what we give" is a true one. Generosity breeds generosity, and contempt breeds contempt. And these are both choices, so the question is, what do we choose? What do we choose in general, and what do we choose specifically in each and every situation? If we want prosperity, or if we want to abandon our fear of financial insecurity, then we have to practice generosity. We have to choose it, not just sometimes, but all of the time.

The generosity-activating question in each life experience is, "What can I give?" We consider what we have to offer and offer it, without question, without complaint, and without expecting anything in return. And the reason for doing this is the way it makes us feel. It makes us feel good! We are participating. We are helping. And our effort, if it is sincere, is appreciated. It's a win-win situation all the way around. Generosity is one of the best feelings there is, and we can make it an ongoing habit in our lives.

If we are not naturally generous or are more naturally suspicious or afraid of others, we can still learn to practice generosity. We can start small. Perhaps we can begin by telling someone that they look nice, by opening a door for one of our elders, by letting someone get in front of us in traffic, or by being pleasant with a cashier. In some basic way, generosity is based on the understanding that we are all in this thing together and doing the best that we can. We all have hard days and dark moods as well as victories and joys. We collectively experience the whole range of human emotions, human realities, and human drama, and not one of us is immune. So it's reasonable to help each other out as we make our way, and it feels good to do so. Whether we are giving help or being helped, the exchange of generosity gives us a sense of well-being, and our sense of well-being is the basis for prosperity in our lives.

Awareness Exercise: Generosity Checklist

By filling out the chart below, you will increase awareness regarding your lifetime practice of generosity, and consequently, your experience of prosperity and well-being. Keep in mind, as you are marking the columns, that "generosity" here is openhearted and willing; it is not a duty-bound and obligatory feeling. It is genuine and compassionate. Consider, as you proceed, whether you are helpful, complimentary, forgiving, thoughtful, considerate, and loving in regard to the individuals listed. Leave any lines blank that do not apply. You will need a pen or a pencil, your journal, and a few minutes of quiet, uninterrupted time.

1. Complete the chart below by putting checkmarks in the appropriate columns:

	Most of the time	Some of the time	Rarely
• I am generous with *myself.*	____	____	____
• I am generous with my *immediate family.*	____	____	____
• I am generous with my *extended family.*	____	____	____
• I am generous with *co-workers.*	____	____	____

+ I am generous
  with *clients*.   ____   ____   ____

+ I am generous
  with *children*.   ____   ____   ____

+ I am generous
  with *older people*.   ____   ____   ____

+ I am generous with
  handicapped people.   ____   ____   ____

+ I am generous
  with *strangers*.   ____   ____   ____

+ I am generous
  with *animals*.   ____   ____   ____

2. Using your journal, take a few minutes to write down
   your reasoning for responding the way you did to the
   chart above. In other words, *how* do you think that your
   behavior exemplifies generosity or a lack thereof in
   relation to yourself and the group listed? Acknowledge
   areas in your life where you might expand and improve
   your generosity and record how you might do that.
   Remember that you can start small.

The act of generosity has a snowball effect. The more generous we are, the more generous we feel, and the more generous

others are with us. Being thoughtful in this way takes us out of ourselves and opens our hearts; and the benefit that we experience is the same or greater than the benefit others receive from our being generous. So it feels good all around. As such, it's a valuable habit to develop, and one that will increase our feelings of well-being from the inside out.

Gratitude

If all of the principles we have discussed to this point are the legs and support beams on the table of prosperity, then gratitude is the table itself. It brings it all together and serves it up. Gratitude is the kingpin principle. It is more than appreciation and more than the understanding of abundance. It is the mastery of recognizing all that we have.

There is an admission, in gratitude, of the priceless and immeasurable reality of our not necessarily deserving what we have, but having it anyway. The blessing of life itself is beyond measure or comprehension, and unexpected gifts galore come from we know not where. Gratitude keeps us humble in that it understands the goodness that befalls us, and the wonder of our own miraculous selves.

Nonetheless, difficult situations arise in life that are emotionally painful and seemingly unfair. If we are living in entitlement rather than gratitude, we are completely dislodged by accidents, sickness, extreme hardship, and death. But from the perspective of a grateful heart, it's possible to see that even our challenges bless us, because it is through them that we learn and grow spiritually. This is the miracle of gratitude. It has transformative power.

As we survive our suffering and come out on the far side of it—out of the darkness and into the light—we come to understand that going through what we go through gives us depth. We become more compassionate of others who are also suffering, and more compassionate with ourselves. Many is the story of individuals who have been through horrific circumstances and live to tell about them. More often than not, they readily admit that what seemed like the worst possible thing at the time actually ended up being the best thing in the end because it changed them and redirected their path. It made them realize what matters and the value of their lives. Most of us have a handful of these experiences in our own history, so we can relate to others when they share their stories with us.

In this way, gratitude is the spiritual principle that is the foundation of our personal evolution. It is a learned understanding that life is fundamentally good, even if it's hard at times, and that if it doesn't kill us, it really does make us stronger. If we are grateful, then we see that everything that happens to us can be construed as a blessing, and it becomes safe to trust in the process of life itself.

Gratitude is a state of being. We say "I am grateful," and thereby acknowledge that it is something that we are. But as with all things in our lives, it's a choice. We can be grateful, or not.

The opposite of grateful is resentful, angry, or bitter—take your pick. By living this way, we are impoverished by our own internal point of view. We see ourselves as victims and life as a kind of punishing game of survival. Life happens to us, and we refuse to learn from it. We wait for the other shoe to drop and the next disaster and the next. We feel certain that others have it better than we do and that there's no such thing as equal opportunity.

Yet, at the most basic level, we are equal. There's no denying that fact. We are equal at the level of our being alive and being human. We have equal opportunity for simple pleasures and sensational wonders, and equal opportunity for suffering. We all experience both ends of the spectrum, and that can't be helped. It's what we do with these things and how we choose to process them that distinguishes our perception of prosperity in life.

If, however, the concept of being grateful for suffering seems an impossible ideal, then we have to approach things more simply to begin. We have to start from wherever we are. We need to develop the habit of gratitude itself and let it grow slowly in our lives. It's a way of looking and a way of seeing. It requires that we raise our awareness enough to acknowledge where we do feel grateful, and further acknowledge that we have plenty to be grateful for, whether we currently think so, or not. Doing this is a practice that we can all benefit from, no matter where we find ourselves on the gratitude-proficiency scale.

Appreciation Exercise: Daily Gratitude List

By making a gratitude list in your journal at first, and eventually as a form of inner commentary, you will raise feelings of prosperity, well-being, and goodness in your life. You can be grateful for anything—small things, big things, material things, spiritual things, people, places, weather, outcomes. There are no limits to what you can feel grateful for. All you need for this exercise is a pen or a pencil, your journal, and a few minutes a day.

1. Write the numbers 1–10 in a column on a blank page in your journal.

2. Put one thing you're grateful for beside each number.

3. Do this every day for a few weeks or more, until it begins to come naturally.

4. When you feel ready, change the habit from a written list to an internal one and continue the exercise as a daily practice.

EXAMPLE

I am grateful for:

1. Hot showers (What a great way to start the day!)

2. Sunshine (It was so delicious through the kitchen window this morning!)

3. Wintertime (Cold air and the smell of wood-smoke is the ultimate combination of refreshment and comfort.)

4. Goose down (Soft and light and warm all at once—delightful!)

5. Weekends (What a pleasure to be able to structure my own time.)

6. Mountain views (They never cease to soothe and inspire me.)

7. Perseverance (This enables me to accomplish anything I set my mind to, bit by bit.)

8. Chickens (I love the way they cluck and coo in the coop.)

9. Laughter (It's so much fun to be silly and enjoy the people I live with.)

10. Love (Where would I be without it? It's the reason for everything!)

In the example, I have detailed my reasoning using parenthesis to show the process of appreciation, but you needn't do that in writing unless you feel particularly inclined. You can keep your lists ultra-simple. The point is to get in the habit of recognizing things that you are grateful for wherever and whenever you find them. They can be small things within your day, spiritual concepts that enrich your life, staples like your health and home, or whatever else you come across. Anything and everything can fit the bill.

Gratitude in Action

It's one thing to verbally acknowledge and identify things that we are grateful for. It's a step in the right direction. But it's not enough. There is another, more important step, and that is to actively demonstrate our gratitude in the way we behave. It's easy to miss out on the benefits of prosperity by skimping on this step. We say that our family is important to us, but we mistreat them by being grouchy and impatient whenever we're home. We say that we are grateful for our job, but we show up late and bad-mouth our employer to our co-workers. We articulate appreciation for our houses and cars, but we don't keep them properly clean and maintained.

These examples and many like them are the missed detail. This is what makes us feel less than prosperous. From a spiritual and energetic perspective, if we are callous, careless, or disrespectful with anything, it means that we hold it in low regard. We are demonstrating through our behavior that we could take it or leave it—that we are not invested and we don't really care. The implication of such behavior is that we are entitled, so we can do as we please.

This thinking is at the root of our dissatisfaction in life. We dishonor what matters and disrespect the things we are blessed with, and then wonder why we feel so out of sorts. Living in this mentally manufactured reality, we lose our proper place and position in the big picture and forget that we are alive by grace and not by right. It's a tragic error on our part, and we suffer for it.

If we value our lives, and the people and things in our lives, we must treat them with care and respect. This is a cyclical principle, and a what-goes-around-comes-around concept. If I want to feel rich, then I have to treat my possessions as treasures. I wouldn't keep priceless artwork in a pile in my garage, so why would I keep anything else that way either? Care is the cornerstone of gratitude, meaning attention, consideration, and respect. This is the moral code of a prosperous individual. Without these things, life becomes a slipshod affair.

To to be prosperous and well, we have to take care of ourselves, our environment, our relationships, and our dreams. Our responsibility is to nurture every aspect of our lives and to recognize our incredible blessings and say thank you in the way that we behave. If we fail to do this, we miss out on prosperity. We sit around passively waiting for well-being to drop in our lap instead of stepping up to meet it.

When we take responsibility for ourselves and our own prosperity, nothing can strip it from us. It's a way of being that translates into a way of behaving. We are rich because we recognize our blessings, and because we take care of what is ours. No amount of money can purchase what we already have.

Appreciation Exercise: Caring for Our Lives

Learning to respect and care for yourself, others, the environment, and your material possessions will make you feel blessed and prosperous from the inside out. You will need willingness and the daily discipline to do the work.

+ Demonstrate gratitude for your physical being by eating well, moving daily, getting enough sleep, and thinking about your body in loving ways.

+ Demonstrate gratitude for your relationships by making time for your friends and family, by being willing to communicate honestly, and by listening to them with your full attention. Make every effort to be nonjudgmental, to show compassion, and to be willing to accept responsibility when you have been wrong, and willing to forgive others when they have wronged you.

+ Demonstrate gratitude for your physical possessions by keeping things neatly organized, well-maintained, clean, and clear of clutter.

+ Demonstrate gratitude for the natural environment by noticing it—by listening for birds, appreciating trees, picking up trash, recycling, using less energy, and spending at least a little time outside every day in the fresh air.

When we live our lives and treat the people and things that we encounter with care and respect, a resulting sense of gratitude emerges. Our lives are sacred, and the more that we honor that truth, the more prosperity we are likely to feel.

Review and Daily Action Plan

Whatever lack of prosperity we may be conditioned to feeling in life is not the result of a lack of prosperity. It is the result of our fears and excess, and a misunderstanding of our purpose. By raising our awareness and increasing our appreciation for who we are and the things that we have, we can learn prosperity consciousness. It already belongs to us, but we have to claim it. We have to become habituated to caring for the things that matter and treating ourselves, others, and the environment with gratitude and respect.

1. Identify fears surrounding financial insecurity and disarm them by thinking them through.

2. Practice the understanding that less is more.

3. Appreciate the real value of things, and what really matters.

4. Create a personal mission statement.

5. Make a commitment to experience abundance and prosperity in life.

6. Eliminate physical clutter.

7. Examine and increase the principle
   of generosity with yourself and others.

8. Make a daily gratitude list.

9. Take loving care of yourself, your relationships,
   and the environment in which you live.

Conclusion

I have recommended a variety of daily practices in each section throughout the book. These are not designed to overwhelm you or make your already-busy life even busier. They are, instead, suggestions for creating new routines that can better serve your desire to feel good. Learning to clarify your convoluted thinking process and quiet your mind, affirming what you want, expressing what you love, being grateful and forgiving, moving your body, living in a technology-free zone for a little bit of time every day, keeping your life and the space you occupy clear of clutter, setting boundaries, and being rigorously self-honest in an ongoing way—these are strategies for good living.

Through the application of effort and the repetitive practice of positive action, you can enjoy a sense of well-being in your life. No matter your circumstances or your situation, happiness is possible. It does not come from things or other people; it comes from inside of you. And you can choose to take responsibility for how you feel, or not. But doing so ensures your evolution and enables your satisfaction, so I highly recommend it.

If you are willing to dedicate the time and the effort that it takes to establish the good habits described and suggested in this book—maybe three months or so of a bit of daily work— then you can become like the cruise ship we described in chapter one. You will hardly notice you're changing at all, until, one day, you realize that you have made a full turn.